How to Protect Your Family's Assets from Devastating
Nursing Home Costs

MEDICAID SECRETS

K. Gabriel Heiser, Attorney

Phylius Press

Phylius Press
464 Blackfoot St., Suite 101
Superior, CO 80027
(303) 447-6855

This publication is designed to provide accurate and authoritative information in regard to the subject matter covered. It is sold with the understanding that the publisher is not engaged in rendering legal, accounting, or other professional service. If legal advice or other expert assistance is required, the services of a competent professional should be sought.

—From a *Declaration of Principles* jointly adopted by a committee of the American Bar Association and a committee of publishers and associations

Published by:

Phylius Press

Phylius Press
464 Blackfoot St., Suite 101
Superior, CO 80027
(303) 447-6855

Library of Congress Control Number: 2006936564

ISBN-13: 978-0-9790801-1-1
ISBN-10: 0-9790801-1-8

For additional copies:
www.MedicaidSecrets.com

ABOUT THE AUTHOR

K. Gabriel Heiser, J.D., of Boulder ElderLaw, has focused exclusively on estate planning and Medicaid eligibility planning, including trusts, estates, gifts, and related tax issues, since graduating from Boston University School of Law in 1983. He also practiced in Massachusetts, where he was Chairman of the Estate Planning Committee of the Massachusetts Bar Association, and in Tennessee, where he was the founder and first Chairman of the Nashville Bar Association's Estate Planning Committee and where he served as President of the Middle Tennessee Planned Giving Council (1997). He is a long-time member of the National Academy of Elder Law Attorneys (NAELA), a Fellow of the American College of Trust and Estate Counsel (ACTEC)—the highest designation for trust and estate attorneys in the U.S.—and is AV® rated by Martindale-Hubbell®, the country's preeminent lawyer peer rating service.

Attorney Heiser is a frequent seminar leader and participant in the areas of estate and gift tax, charitable gifts and trusts, Medicaid eligibility planning, and sophisticated estate planning. He has taught as a member of the Adjunct Faculty of the College for Financial Planning at David Lipscomb University, as an instructor in Estate Planning Law (1996-1998), and has been certified as an Estate Planning Law Specialist by The Estate Law Specialist Board, Inc., the only American Bar Association-accredited program for certification of an attorney as an estate planning specialist.*

Fellow, American College of Trust and Estate Counsel (ACTEC): Being elected to ACTEC is one of the highest honors an estate planning attorney can receive. ACTEC is a non-profit association composed of approximately 2,700 of the most accomplished estate planning practitioners in the United States and Canada. A lawyer cannot apply for membership in the College; Fellows of the College are nominated by other Fellows in their geographic area and are elected by the membership at large. To qualify for membership, a lawyer must have at least 10 years of experience in the active

---

* Colorado does not certify attorneys as specialists in any field.
  Author photo by Karen Hartman.

practice of probate and trust law or estate planning. Lawyers and law professors are elected to be Fellows by the other members, based on their outstanding professional reputation, exceptional skill, and substantial contributions to the field by lecturing, writing, teaching and participating in bar activities.

Member: Boulder Estate Planning Council, National Academy of Elder Law Attorneys, Boulder Bar Association (Tax, Estate Planning, and Probate Section), Colorado Bar Association (Elder Law Section).

AV® rated: Attorney Heiser is proud to have received an **AV® rating* from Martindale-Hubbell®**, the country's preeminent lawyer rating service. An AV rating is a significant accomplishment—a testament to the fact that a lawyer's peers rank him at the highest level of professional excellence. A lawyer must be admitted to the bar for 10 years or more to receive an AV rating. His AV rating is based on peer reviews by members of the Bar and Judiciary. That means that the lawyers and judges with whom he has worked closely feel that he is among the best in the business not only for his legal skills, but also for his honesty, integrity and ethics.

Author: Retirement Plan Distributions: The Rules (Boulder Estate Planning Council presentation, 2/21/06); **Co-author:** Estate Planning in Tennessee (Lorman Education Services, 2000); Key Issues in Estate Planning and Probate (National Business Institute, 2000); Sophisticated Estate Planning Strategies for the Advanced Practitioner in Tennessee (National Business Institute, 1998), Advanced Estate Planning Techniques in Tennessee (National Business Institute, 1997), Family Limited Partnerships in Tennessee (National Business Institute, 1996), Living Trusts and Other Estate Planning Alternatives in Tennessee (National Business Institute, 1995), Estate Planning for the Elder and Disabled Client (Nashville Bar Association, 1994).

www.MedicaidSecrets.com/blog
Explore attorney Heiser's *Elder Law Blog!* This daily diary of elder law and estate planning topics will be of great interest to readers of *Medicaid Secrets*. Submit questions or suggestions for additional topics by registering on the blog page.

*"AV" is a registered certification mark of Reed Elsevier Properties Inc., used in accordance with the Martindale-Hubbell certification procedures, standards and policies.

SUMMARY OF CONTENTS

TABLE OF CONTENTS

Chapter 1

INTRODUCTION

You are reading this book because you already know the cold, hard fact: nursing homes are expensive, and without careful planning, a stay in one can easily bankrupt all but the most affluent families. Considering that the average cost of a nursing home in the U.S. is $6,250 a month, you're looking at a bill of over $375,000 for your family member with Alzheimer's disease, whose nursing home stay typically is five years or more.

What most people don't realize is that, unless you have private long-term care insurance, the government will only pay the nursing home bill if your cash is below $2,000. Medicare will only cover you for a maximum of 100 days, if they cover you at all; Social Security won't cover these bills, either. Only Medicaid will cover you.

This book will explain in plain English what the rules are and how you can qualify for Medicaid coverage of your nursing home bills yet still protect your life savings.

This book covers the federal Medicaid rules for single individuals (never married, divorced, or widowed) as well as married couples. It will discuss both the income limits and asset limits. It will explain what you can do—to protect your assets and not get in trouble or be penalized—and what you cannot do.

It will cover the significant changes that resulted from the enactment of the federal Deficit Reduction Act of 2005 (referred to as the "DRA"), which became law on February 8, 2006.

Without proper legal advice, you will undoubtedly be told that you must spend down your assets until you have reduced your life savings to the point that you qualify for Medicaid coverage of your nursing home bills. Unfortunately, this leaves you without the cash to pay for items and "extras" not paid for by the Medicaid program. What if your family wants to visit you and you'd like to pay their way? What if you want some new clothes? A large-screen TV? Remote headphones so you can hear your TV better? Specialized or alternative medical treatments not covered by Medicaid? Without some source of private funds, you will be at the mercy of the Medicaid program. If they don't pay for it, you're simply out of luck.

Also, most people with children would prefer to be able to pass on at least part of their life savings—and hopefully the family home—to their children. And many people without children would still prefer to give their assets either to other family members—siblings, nieces, nephews—or their church, synagogue or other charitable or educational institution, than to use up every dime of their life savings paying for their last years in a nursing home.

It is important to note that, while all the advice given in this book is completely legal, some techniques may not work in all states. The reason for this is that the Medicaid system, while based on federal law, allows each state to select certain optional rules. Accordingly, the Medicaid rules reflect a crazy patchwork quilt of federal rules, regulations, and cases, and state statutes, regulations, and case law. As if that weren't bad enough, what may be approved in one county— or even by one caseworker within a single county—may not fly in a different county or by a different caseworker. Sometimes the decisions of the caseworker will be wrong, and you will need to appeal to a higher level supervisor, or even request a mini-trial known as a

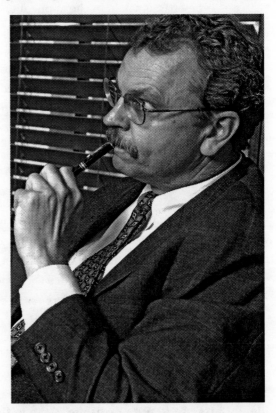

"Fair Hearing." The point is that you cannot simply take the information here at face value without checking with a local elder law attorney who is familiar with your state's Medicaid rules. But **after reading this book you will know what to ask the attorney and you will have some idea what is in store for your family.**

How to Use This Book

As you can see from the introduction, the Medicaid system is extremely complex. Your facts and circumstances will differ from those of everyone else in the following ways:

- Age, health, and life expectancy of the potential Medicaid applicant
- Marital status of the applicant
- If married, the age, health, and life expectancy of the potential Medicaid applicant's husband or wife
- Type of assets held in the applicant's name
  - Is there a home? A family farm?
  - Family business?
  - IRAs or other retirement accounts?
  - Pensions or Social Security income?
- Total amount of assets held in the applicant's name
- Number of children in the applicant's family
- Family dynamics
- Location of various family members
- Other unique factors

Every example given in this book may not apply to your particular situation. As stated above, the laws of your state may not permit a specific technique discussed in the book. In addition, the laws, rules, and regulations may have changed in your state since the time this was written. In particular, the recently enacted federal DRA has yet to be fully phased in, in most states. Thus, we are in a transition period, further complicating matters.

As a result, the only sure way to know what will work, and what is best for your particular situation, is to consult an elder law attorney (see *How to Find the Right Kind of Attorney*, in the Appendix (page 189)). In other words, **do not attempt to put any of the ideas in this book into place without the assistance of a specialist elder law attorney! To do otherwise is to risk your life savings.**

While this book won't replace the need to consult with an experienced elder law attorney, it will tell you what you need to know to make sure you are getting good advice. You will be on firm ground when you consult with an attorney and will have a good idea if the attorney really knows what he or she is talking about.

Thus, the best way to use this book is as an **Idea Book**. It can stimulate your thinking and arm you with lots of great ideas and concepts to bring to your attorney. It will educate you on both the basic concepts of the Medicaid system as it applies to anyone living in a nursing home as well as more advanced asset protection techniques. And, most importantly, it can keep you from making mistakes. Once you become aware of the planning possibilities available to you, hopefully, you will steer clear of making the kinds of transfers or blunders that can get you in trouble down the road!

As you read through the book, check off or highlight any ideas that you think may apply to your particular situation. Discuss them with your family members and finally bring them to the attention of your attorney. Your attorney can then evaluate them in light of your state's laws as well as the financial and health status of the family member who is planning on applying for Medicaid coverage.

Is It Legal?

Have no fears—every technique and option discussed in this book is 100% legal! As an attorney for over 23 years, I would never suggest any planning technique or option that is not legal. For example, simply "hiding" money is not an option: to do so and not report the asset on a Medicaid application is clearly a fraud against the state and federal governments, with severe legal consequences. There are ample ways to achieve your goals using completely legal methods. Don't risk going to jail or incurring huge fines and penalties by doing anything illegal!

Is It Ethical?

Some people simply do not like the fact that there are attorneys who specialize in advising clients how to save their money and qualify for Medicaid coverage sooner. Their theory is that Medicaid is a "welfare" program for the poor, broke, and destitute, and was not designed as a way for middle class parents to pass their money on to their children at taxpayer expense.

My answer to this is as follows:

John Jones lives next door to Sam Smith. Both of these fine fellows are age 75 and have about $100,000 in the bank and a home that is paid off. John has a friend named Joe who lives across town in an apartment, who used to have some savings but who squandered it on drink and gambling.

John has a heart attack and is rushed to the hospital. Thank goodness he survives, but the operation costs $80,000. Lucky for him he's covered by Medicare, so he arrives home with his life savings intact. Upon his death, his $100,000 and his home pass to his children, under his will.

Meanwhile, Sam has a stroke and has to be moved to a nursing home. Since the nursing home costs $8,000 a month, Sam's life savings are gone in about a year. At that point, Sam qualifies for Medicaid, which pays his nursing home bills. He continues to reside in the nursing home for two more years, and upon his death the state has spent another $200,000 on his care. Under federal law, the state must be repaid at Sam's death, and since the only asset in his name is his house, it has to be sold to repay the state, leaving his heirs almost nothing.

As for Joe, his drinking takes its toll, and he also winds up in a nursing home. Since he is broke, he immediately qualifies for Medicaid, which pays all his bills. Upon his death, the state cannot be repaid since Joe leaves no estate.

So, in essence, the government is content to pay all of John's hospital bills but wants Sam to first impoverish himself and then they take his house at his death, to pay for his nursing home bills. Meanwhile, Joe is rewarded for his profligate lifestyle by getting a free ride from the government; his family does not have to chip in one penny for his care.

Oh—there's one more guy we need to meet: Bob, who also managed to save up $100,000 and pay off his house, but who was a little more thoughtful than Sam and who hired an elder law attorney to give him advice. That lawyer was aware of all the provisions of the Medicaid rules and regulations, and advised Bob to make some loans, some approved purchases, and some gifts to family members, so that by the time Bob entered a nursing home, his assets were protected. Thus, Bob received the same care as Sam, but his assets were passed to his family and did not have to be spent on nursing home bills.

Is Sam, who managed to build up a small amount of savings, more ethical than Joe, who squandered his money and then had the government pay for his care? Is Sam more ethical than Bob, who simply followed the rules and regulations enacted by the state and federal government, and managed to protect his life savings and house? And how does that differ from the guy in the Lexus who pays top dollar to the Big Four accounting firm for clever tax planning, setting up offshore corporations so his business can legally avoid paying millions in income taxes? Legal, yes. Ethical? I leave that to you. But in any event, is it any more ethical than Medicaid planning?

As the great Judge Learned Hand famously said in the case of *Helvering v. Gregory* (1934),

> *"Any one may so arrange his affairs that his taxes shall be as low as possible; he is not bound to choose that pattern which will best pay the Treasury; there is not even a patriotic duty to increase one's taxes. . . . Over and over again courts have said that there is nothing sinister in so arranging one's affairs as to keep taxes as low as possible. Everybody does so, rich or poor; and all do right, for nobody owes any public duty to pay more than the law demands: taxes are enforced exactions, not voluntary contributions. To demand more in the name of morals is mere cant."*

The United States Supreme Court reinforced this sentiment in affirming the above ruling:

> *"The legal right of a taxpayer to decrease the amount of what otherwise would be his taxes, or altogether avoid them, by means which the law permits, cannot be doubted."*

No one says you have to take advantage of every possible available legal planning technique if you don't want to. You can also decide not to claim, say, a charitable deduction that is legally available to you on your Form 1040 and pay more income tax than you are required to do. **But it is certainly not unethical simply to avail yourself of the laws as they were enacted by the government in order to minimize your expenditures on nursing home care, and pass those savings on to your children.** This book will show you exactly how you can do that.

Chapter 2

WHAT IS "MEDICAID"?

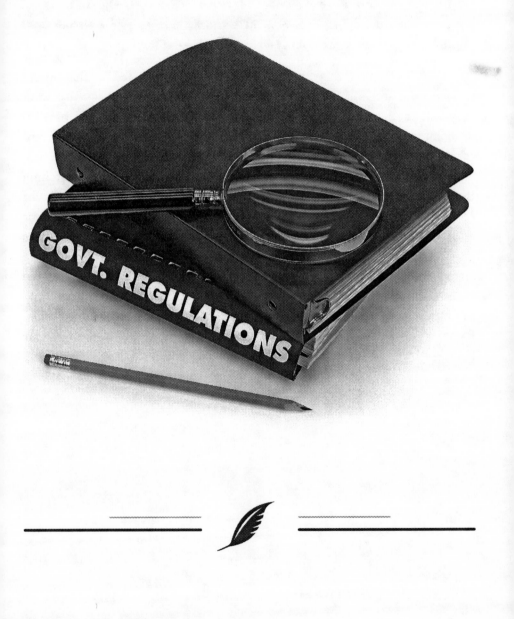

In brief,

> Medicaid is a joint federal-state program for the medical care of
> certain needy populations within the United States. Although
> established by federal law, the Medicaid program is for the most
> part administered by the individual states. The cost is shared
> by the federal government and the states, with the federal
> government paying between 50% and 83% of the cost (it pays
> more to poorer states, less to the wealthier states).

What makes this area of the law so complicated is that under
the federal statutes there are many options given to the states as to what
they will pay for and who is entitled to coverage. As a result, you have 50
different versions of the Medicaid rules, with each state selecting a different
combination of options, and each one interpreting the same laws differently.
That leaves the residents of each state (including the lawyers, there!) scratching
their heads trying to figure out what they can and cannot do, to qualify for
Medicaid coverage. Unfortunately, you cannot simply ask the government for
an advance ruling or interpretation, like you can with the IRS. That forces
you to try something first and hope for the best. If you're challenged by the
state Medicaid authorities, you can appeal their interpretation if you disagree
with it, and even take them to court. Of course, very few people are willing
to do that, because of the significant expense and hassle involved in such a
lawsuit. So that leaves you relying on your best guess of what you—and your
lawyer—think the state rules actually are.

Chapter 3

WHAT IS COVERED BY "MEDICAID"?

Medical Coverage

Once you have been approved for Medicaid, virtually all of your medical bills will be paid by the program. This includes your prescription drugs, hospital stays, nursing care, etc. Medicare may overlap this coverage, but one way or another your medical bills will be paid for you. Those who are receiving both Medicaid *and* Medicare coverage are known as "dual eligibles." Prescription drugs, formerly paid for by Medicaid, will now be paid for by Medicare Part D.

The following services *must* be offered by all states:

- inpatient hospital services
- outpatient hospital services
- physician services
- medical and surgical dental services
- nursing facility services for individuals age 21 or older
- home health care for persons eligible for nursing facility services
- lab and x-ray services
- family nurse practitioner services

The following services are *optional*, but most states will offer them, also:

- ambulatory services to individuals entitled to institutional care
- home health services to individuals entitled to nursing facility services
- prescribed drug coverage
- optometrist services and eyeglasses
- prosthetic devices
- dental services
- in-home assistance

Care in Your Home

If you are living in your home, i.e., not in a nursing home, the Medicaid program refers to you as living "in the community," and Medicaid will still pay for certain services if you qualify. Many states have a program called "HCBS," which stands for "Home and Community Based Services." Until recently, a state wishing to provide Medicaid assistance to elderly people outside the nursing home had to apply to the federal government for a specific "waiver" of the usual Medicaid rules. But beginning in 2007, all states will be eligible to offer this program *without* first having to obtain a federal waiver. Hopefully, this will expand the access to HCBS nationally. In any event, you must check to see if your state currently offers this program to its residents or plans to do so shortly.

In general, HCBS will pay for the following in-home services:

- case management
- personal care services
- respite care services (i.e., care for the patient in a nursing home for a few days, to give the home caregiver a needed break)
- adult day health services
- homemaker/home health aide services
- habilitation (i.e., assists people in furthering their skills in the areas of mobility, social behaviors, self care, basic safety, housekeeping, personal hygiene, health care, and financial management)

Beginning in 2007, states may begin to offer to those who are already in a nursing home the option of living in the community, allowing them the ability to interact with their family and community away from the institutional setting. They will be able to have the same level of care, and be covered by Medicaid. Be sure to check if your state has implemented this new program or plans to do so shortly.

Assisted Living

In most states, it is possible to have Medicaid pay for certain services even if you are living in an assisted living facility. These are under the HCBS program described above. Note that the facility must be "Medicaid certified," so you will want to make sure about that when you are searching for a facility to move into. Note, however, that the facility's cost of basic room and board will *not* be paid for by Medicaid, as it would be if you resided in a nursing home.

Nursing Homes

Medicaid will pay the full nursing home bill, including room, board, and all nursing care costs.

However, it is very important to note that although 58% of all nursing home beds are filled with patients on the Medicaid program, not every nursing home accepts Medicaid payments. Thus, it is **extremely important** that you find out before you sign up for a nursing home whether it accepts Medicaid patients. While it is against the law for a nursing home to evict you because you run out of money and must go from private pay to Medicaid, that does not apply if the nursing home does not accept Medicaid from anyone! Be sure to ask! It is very upsetting to the nursing home resident to have to relocate from one nursing home to another, after finally accepting the fact that they are in a nursing home for good, have gotten used to the routines, made friends, become acquainted with the nurses, etc.

Chapter 4

APPLYING FOR BENEFITS

When to Apply

Applying Too Late

Applying too late can mean that the opportunity to have the government pay for your family member's care will be lost, costing your family thousands of dollars. Although it is permissible to apply for benefits for the period starting up to three months prior to the date of application, you cannot go back any further than that (see Retroactive Coverage on the next page). Thus, it makes sense to apply as soon as you are sure your family member can qualify.

Applying Too Early

Applying too early can be a very expensive mistake if gifts have been made that affect eligibility! Most gifts made by the Medicaid applicant and/or spouse can cause a period of disqualification if either or both of them apply for Medicaid within three to five years of the gift (depending on the date made; see *Transferring Assets*, page 49, for a detailed explanation). Applying before this "lookback period" (see page 54) has expired can cause a huge increase in the penalty period (see page 50).

Example:

John makes a transfer to his children on March 1, 2006, of his house, worth $250,000. If he waits until March 1, 2011 to apply for Medicaid, there will be no period of disqualification, because his gift was made outside of the five-year lookback period. However, if he applies for Medicaid on February 1, 2011, he could be disqualified from receiving Medicaid coverage for 50 months or more (depending on what state he lives in)!

Sometimes it makes sense to apply during the lookback period because you want to get the penalty period running. This technique is explained in more detail below, under the *Half-A-Loaf* discussion, page 130.

So the rule is, never apply until you're sure your family member qualifies, OR if you are certain you want the penalty period to start immediately. In any event, if any gifts have been made within the last five years, the opinion of an experienced elder law attorney should be sought prior to actually applying for Medicaid, to make sure the time is right to do so.

Where to Apply

Every state will have a system in place to permit you to apply for Medicaid benefits. The best way to find out where you need to go is to consult the *State Medicaid Agency Contacts* list in the *Appendix* of this book (page 215).

List of State Agencies

For a list of state agencies that supervise the application process, see the *State Medicaid Agency Contacts* list in the *Appendix* of this book (page 215).

Application Process

The application form will require you to list your current income and assets. You will also need to bring in your bank account records going back anywhere from 6 months to as much as five years. You may have to provide copies of deeds, trusts, and insurance policies. Thus, it is a good idea to start gathering the necessary information in advance of your application. Otherwise, your inability to provide the necessary documents or information could cause a delay in the processing of your application, which in turn could cause you to lose valuable benefits.

Retroactive Coverage

It is possible to apply for Medicaid coverage for a period beginning up to three months prior to the date of application. If the applicant *would have* qualified for Medicaid as of such date had he or she applied at such time, then the applicant will be covered starting on such date. (A state may even cover the applicant as of the first day of that month.) For example, if you thought you would not qualify for Medicaid for several months and then found out you actually *could have* qualified, you can apply for Medicaid immediately, and ask for coverage going back up to three months. Unfortunately, the period of time before the three-month date will not be covered by Medicaid, even if you could have qualified had you applied back then. Thus it is very important to apply as soon as you are qualified; once that three-month retroactive window closes, your family may wind up having to pay privately for your care when you *could* have gotten Medicaid to pay all of your nursing home expenses.

Documentation of Citizenship

Beginning July 1, 2006, anyone applying for or receiving Medicaid will need to prove that they are either a U.S. citizen or national, or a qualified alien. Such proof must be made at the time of applying for Medicaid for the first time, or upon the first redetermination of eligibility (which is done once a year following initial approval) for those already receiving Medicaid coverage. It is only done once per person.

Such proof may only be made by one or more of the following:

- U.S. passport
- Certificate of Naturalization (Form N-550 or N-570)
- Certificate of U. S. Citizenship (Form N-560 or N-561)
- A valid state-issued driver's license or i.d. document BUT ONLY if the state requires proof of U.S. citizenship prior to issuance or obtains and verifies the individual's Social Security Number
- If none of the above is available, then the applicant can provide any of the following to establish citizenship:
  - U.S. birth certificate
  - Other evidence of U.S. citizenship if born abroad, adopted, etc.
- If none of the above is available, there are still other methods allowed, in rare circumstances, such as hospital records, census records, medical records, and written affidavit if all else fails.
- If one of the first four methods listed above cannot be used, then the applicant must also submit one of the following to establish identity:
  - A valid state-issued driver's license with photo or other identifying information
  - School i.d. card with photo
  - U.S. military card or draft record
  - Government i.d. card with photo or other i.d. information
  - Etc.

- All copies must either be originals or copies certified by the issuing agency; notarized copies are not acceptable.
- Such other documentation as the Secretary of Health and Human Services may allow, by regulation. As of this writing, there is only an "interim final rule" from the Center for Medicare and Medicaid (CMS).

Because it may take some time to obtain the above documentation, particularly if one of the first four methods of proof is unavailable, the family should assist the prospective Medicaid applicant in getting this documentation together as soon as possible.

Nursing Home Bills During the Application Period

Once you apply for Medicaid, the nursing home where you are staying may not make you pay the nursing home bill until the application process is complete and you are determined to be ineligible to receive Medicaid. If you are approved, then the nursing home will be able to apply to Medicaid for the back charges. If you are denied and then appeal the denial, the nursing home may be able to charge you during the period of the appeal process, but if you are ultimately approved for Medicaid, the nursing home will have to refund to your family all the fees it received from your family during the appeals process.

Since it can be difficult and time-consuming to get the nursing home to refund money you already paid them, you should always hold off on paying them during the initial application period. Remember, you are not responsible for paying the nursing home during this period—by law, they have to wait.

Chapter 5

MEDICAL QUALIFICATION RULES

In addition to the strict financial rules that are the focus of this book, there are also medical qualifications to meet before a person will be eligible for Medicaid coverage. The applicant must prove he or she is at least age 65, blind, or disabled. According to the federal regulations, to be disabled means that you are unable "to do any substantial gainful activity by reason of any medically determinable physical or mental impairment that can be expected to result in death or which has lasted or can be expected to last for a continuous period of not less than 12 months."

Typically, the state will send a nurse or trained intake worker to the Medicaid applicant's home, to interview the applicant. The nurse or worker will have a checklist of Activities of Daily Living (ADLs) and in order to be deemed "sick" enough to qualify for Medicaid, the applicant must "fail" a certain number of these tests. Thus, this is not a time for the applicant to downplay his or her disabilities; such comments can cause the nurse or worker to think the applicant is actually in better shape than he or she really is, with the result that Medicaid coverage will be denied. If that happens, the applicant's only recourse at that point is an expensive appeals process.

Meeting the medical qualifications is not typically an issue when you are looking at a frail elderly or Alzheimer's patient. The real issues are more often that of having too much income or too many assets, so let's move on and take a detailed look at that.

Chapter 6

INCOME QUALIFICATION RULES

Unmarried

An unmarried individual may not have more than $1,869 of income per month. (This 2007 figure, published by the federal government, changes annually to reflect cost-of-living changes.) "Income" for these purposes includes both "earned" income (wages) and "unearned" income (interest and dividends).

What if your income exceeds this amount? There are actually two different ways this is handled, depending on the state in which you live.

Income-cap States

In an "income-cap" state, if your income is even one dollar above the limit, you are initially disqualified from Medicaid. (At the time of this writing, the following are "income-cap" states: AL, AK, CO, DE, ID, MS, NE, NM, SC, SD, TN, and WY.) A problem arises if you earn too much money to qualify for Medicaid to help you pay the nursing home bill, but not enough to pay for it privately! It was this exact dilemma that led to the lawsuit that finally created the solution: All these states now allow you to set up a simple trust and have your income paid to the trust. The trust then takes the income and pays it to the nursing home each month. A family member can act as the trustee of this trust, keeping the costs down. Assuming you follow some basic rules about this process, your excess income will not prevent you from qualifying for Medicaid, *unless* your income exceeds the amount that Medicaid would otherwise pay to the nursing home each month for your care.

This type of trust is known as a "Qualified Income Trust" or "Miller Trust" (after the case, *Miller v. Ibarra*, discussed above, that established this trust procedure).

Check to see if your state publishes a standard, short-form trust that is essentially a "fill-in-the-blanks" document. Using such a form means you don't have to hire an attorney to create this trust document for you.

In each of the following examples, assume that the individual applying for Medicaid is single, is already in a nursing home, and has minimal assets.

Example 1:

Sam has only his Social Security income of $900/month to live on. He will qualify for Medicaid. Each month his Social Security check goes to the nursing home, and Medicaid picks up the balance of his bill.

Example 2:

Martin has Social Security income of $1,200 and a small monthly pension of $700. He will also qualify for Medicaid, but since his total income of $1,900 exceeds $1,809 (the income upper limit to avoid needing a trust), a Qualified Income Trust will have to be set up to receive the $1,900 each month. That income is then paid over to the nursing home, and once again Medicaid will pay the balance of the bill.

Example 3:

Mary has Social Security, a pension, and some oil lease income that together total $6,000 per month. In the state where Mary lives, that's actually more than the cost of her monthly nursing home bill, so she will not qualify for Medicaid because her income is just too high. Is there a way for her to reduce her income? She is unable to assign her Social Security or pension to another family member, since those are non-assignable under the law. However, she can probably assign her oil lease interest, which would carry the income with it to the new owner. Of course, such assignment is a gift and will cause a penalty period (see discussion of gifts, page 49). However, it is an option that should be considered and discussed with the elder law attorney who will assist Mary to qualify for Medicaid.

Spenddown States

The balance of the states permit the nursing home resident to spend down his or her monthly income (on medical expenses and, most of these states provide, on nursing home costs), with Medicaid paying the shortfall. In other words, so long as the income of the applicant is below the actual cost of the nursing home, the applicant can qualify for Medicaid (assuming the applicant also meets the asset test).

Married

The treatment of income of a married couple is vastly more complicated than that of a single individual. That is because of the various attribution rules that permit the income of the nursing home spouse to be shifted to the spouse still residing in the community (i.e., the "Community Spouse"). As a result of this opportunity, there is much planning that can be done to maximize the income of the Community Spouse and minimize the income of the nursing home spouse.

> The first rule to remember about the treatment of income when one spouse of a married couple applies for Medicaid is "the name on the check determines whose income it is." So a payment of annuity or pension income to one spouse is deemed that spouse's income only.

If you and your spouse own property jointly, then any income from that property will be deemed to be earned by each spouse 50/50. This also applies to joint bank accounts, payments from a trust, or a promissory note or annuity payable to both spouses. Note that this is a rebuttable presumption: if indeed all of the money in the joint account can be traced to one spouse, then it may be possible to prove that the account income should only be deemed to be that of the contributing spouse.

> The important point to remember is that if you are living in the community and your spouse is in the nursing home, you will not have to contribute any portion of your income toward your spouse's nursing home bill, under the Medicaid rules.

Example:

Joe, who is still living at home, has pension and Social Security income totaling $2,500/month. His wife, Edie, now resides in a nursing home. Her income is only from Social Security and equals only $450/month. Nonetheless, Joe does *not* have to contribute one penny to Edie's nursing home care, once she is approved for Medicaid, and he can keep his entire $2,500 each month.

Although the Community Spouse never has to contribute any of his or her income to the other spouse's care, it is possible for the nursing home spouse's income to be paid to the Community Spouse. So it's a one-way street: income only flows—if at all—*from* the nursing home spouse *to* the Community Spouse, and never vice versa.

That's because the Community Spouse is entitled to a minimum monthly income of $1,650 (this figure is set by the federal government and changes annually, on July 1 of each year). This figure is known as the "Minimum Monthly Maintenance Needs Allowance" or "MMMNA." If the Community Spouse's income is less than the MMMNA, then a certain amount of the nursing home spouse's income may be allocated to the nursing home spouse, sufficient (to the extent possible) to increase the Community Spouse's income up to the MMMNA. Such allotment of income from the nursing home spouse to the Community Spouse is called the Monthly Income Allowance, or MIA.

Example 1:

Assume the Community Spouse has no income other than $500 a month from Social Security, and the nursing home spouse has Social Security of $1,000 a month. Based on these numbers, the amount of the nursing home spouse's income that can be shifted over to the Community Spouse—the MIA—will be $1,000. The Community Spouse will be entitled to keep all the couple's combined income, because the total of their combined income would be only $1,500 per month.Since that's less than the minimum entitlement income of $1,650, the Community Spouse can keep *all* of the income, and Medicaid will pay the entire nursing home bill.

MMMNA	$1,650
Community Spouse's income	(500)
Shortfall	1,150
Nursing home spouse's income	1,000
Amount able to be shifted (MIA)	1,000

NOTE: You can never shift *more* than the shortfall figure, or if less, the total amount of the nursing home spouse's income. If the nursing home spouse's income is less than the shortfall amount, it will be possible to increase the amount of excluded assets the Community Spouse can retain. See CSRA discussion, below.

Example 2:

Assume the Community Spouse has income of $500 a month, and the nursing home spouse has income of $2,000 a month. Based on these numbers, the Community Spouse will be allowed to keep $1,150 from the nursing home spouse's income, i.e., an MIA of $1,150 (which brings the Community Spouse up to $1,650). The nursing home spouse will then contribute the balance of his or her income ($2,000 - $1,150 = $850) every month toward the nursing home bill. Medicaid will pick up the balance of the bill.

MMMNA	$1,650
Community Spouse's income	(500)
Shortfall	1,150
Nursing home spouse's income	2,000
Amount able to be shifted (MIA)	1,150

NOTE: You can never shift *more* than the shortfall figure.

Example 3:

Assume the Community Spouse has income of $2,000 a month, and the nursing home spouse has income of $500 a month. In this case, because the Community Spouse's income exceeds the MMMNA of $1,650, no portion of the nursing home spouse's income is allowed to be shifted to the Community Spouse. As a result, the nursing home spouse must pay all of his or her monthly income toward the nursing home bill, and Medicaid will pick up the balance of the bill, once the nursing home spouse has qualified for Medicaid coverage.

MMMNA	$1,650
Community Spouse's income	(2,000)
Shortfall	-0-
Nursing home spouse's income	500
Amount able to be shifted (MIA)	-0-

Increasing the MMMNA

Sometimes it is possible to increase the income of the Community Spouse above the minimum amount (MMMNA). The advantage of doing so is that more of the couple's total income can be retained by the Community Spouse and less will have to be paid over to the nursing home.

There are three ways to do this: increase the MMMNA by the amount of the Excess Shelter Allowance, apply for a Fair Hearing, or obtain a court order of support for the Community Spouse.

Excess Shelter Allowance (ESA)

If the "shelter" costs of the Community Spouse exceed 30% of the MMMNA, then this excess may be added on top of the MMMNA, but only up to the maximum monthly allowance figure published by the federal government (currently $2,541). Since the current MMMNA is $1,650, 30% of that is $495. So if the shelter costs of the Community Spouse exceed $495, that excess amount may be added to the MMMNA when trying to figure out how much of the nursing home spouse's income can be shifted over to the Community Spouse.

For these purposes, "shelter" expenses only include rent or mortgage payment, condo fees (if any), real estate taxes and homeowner's insurance, and either the standard utility allowance (currently between $198 and $546, depending on the state) or, if your state does not use such an allowance, the actual cost of utilities (heat, electricity, gas). Some states even permit you to use the higher of the standard utility allowance or actual cost of utilities when calculating whether or not you qualify for the Excess Shelter Allowance. Once again, you need to check your own state's regulations on this point.

Example:

Mary lives at home in the community, and her husband, Joe, is in the nursing home. Mary's income is $750 a month, all from Social Security. Joe's monthly income is $2,500, from his Social Security and pension. Because Mary's income is less than $1,650, we know she is entitled to shift a portion of Joe's income to her. Ignoring shelter costs, she is entitled to $1,650 - $750, or $900.

MMMNA	$1,650
Community Spouse's income	(750)
Shortfall	900
Nursing home spouse's income	2,500
Amount able to be shifted (MIA)	900

NOTE: You can never shift *more* than the shortfall figure.

Because Joe has excess income even after he shifts some of it to Mary, we should try to see if there's a way to increase the amount Mary is entitled to. After all, Joe's income will all have to go to the nursing home, where it won't do him any good: it will simply reduce the amount that Medicaid would otherwise pay the nursing home.

So the next step is to see if Mary would be entitled to more of Joe's income if her shelter costs are high enough. Here are the figures:

Condo fees	$250
Real estate taxes	150
Homeowner's insurance	100
Standard Utility Allowance	374
TOTAL:	$874
Shelter allowance	(495)
Excess Shelter Allowance	$379

Because her shelter costs ($874) exceed the permitted standard shelter allowance ($495), Mary is allowed to add the excess ($874 -$495 = $379) to the MMMNA ($1,650) for an increased MMMNA of $2,029 ($1,650 + $379). Since her own income is $750, this means she is entitled to shift $1,279 ($2,029 – $750) from Joe's income to herself, each month. Joe's contribution to the nursing home each month will now be reduced by $1,279. This process allows Mary to keep an additional $15,348 of Joe's income each year!

SUMMARY:

MMMNA	$1,650
Excess Shelter Allowance (ESA)	379
Increased MMMNA	2,029
Community Spouse's income	(750)
Shortfall	1,279
Nursing home spouse's income	2,500
Amount able to be shifted (MIA)	1,279

Family Allowance

An additional amount may be deducted from the nursing home spouse's income before paying the nursing home, if certain other family members are living in the home with the Community Spouse. For these purposes, the term "family member" only includes minor or dependent children, dependent parents, or dependent siblings of the nursing home spouse or of the Community Spouse who are residing with the Community Spouse. To calculate this, you subtract the income of the family member from the MMMNA and divide by three. This amount will be deducted from the nursing home spouse's income and paid over to the Community Spouse for the benefit of the family member. This payment does not count as part of the MMMNA, however, so it is not subject to the MMMNA cap of $2,541.

Fair Hearings

In cases where even the maximum MMMNA is not enough to cover the essential monthly living expenses of the Community Spouse, you can ask for a Fair Hearing before the state Medicaid agency. A Fair Hearing is an administrative appeal within the Medicaid state agency that makes the determination of financial eligibility for Medicaid. It is usually an informal proceeding, but it is a good idea to bring an attorney with you.

For example, the Community Spouse may have unusually high living expenses, very high prescription drug costs, or a dependent relative living with him with expenses that exceed the family allowance. If he is successful at the Fair Hearing, he will be permitted to shift a greater amount of income from the nursing home spouse to himself each month.

The test is whether the Community Spouse needs income above even the maximum MMMNA, "due to exceptional circumstances resulting in significant financial duress."

For example, if the Community Spouse lives in assisted living or at home with full-time home health care, the costs can easily exceed $4,000 per month. In such a case, there is a good argument for an increased MMMNA, and a Fair Hearing would be the way to do this.

Court Order of Support

If the maximum MMMNA is still insufficient to meet the monthly income needs of the Community Spouse, the Community Spouse can petition the local court for an Order of Support. The Order will set forth the amount of income that the nursing home spouse must pay each month to the Community Spouse. This Order must be recognized by the Medicaid agency. The petition to the court should be done prior to applying for Medicaid, but may be done before or after the "resource assessment" (see *Snapshot Rule*, page 42).

Chapter 7

ASSET QUALIFICATION RULES

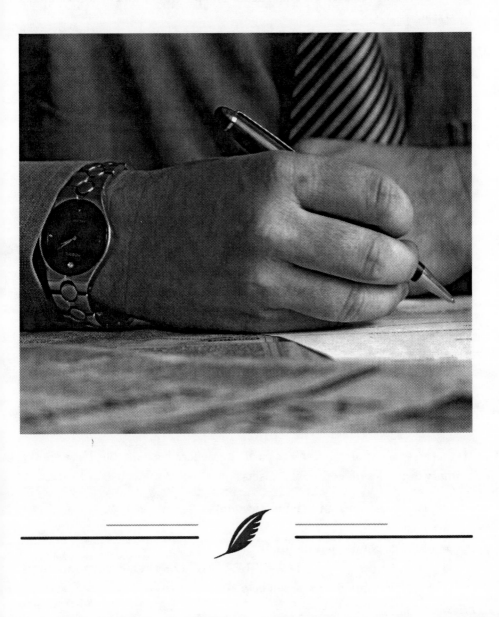

What's Counted, What's Excluded?

Although there are strict limits as to how much money and other assets a person or married couple may have in order to qualify for Medicaid, not all assets will count against the Medicaid applicant. Certain assets are countable, some are deemed unavailable, and others are specifically excluded by statute.

In determining if one spouse of a married couple can qualify for Medicaid, the couple must consider all assets of *both* spouses, whether owned separately or jointly, according to the rules below, and then determine if they are countable, unavailable, or excluded. The Community Spouse will then be able to "protect" a certain amount of the countable assets, as more fully explained at *Married,* page 42).

Valuation

In determining what value your various assets have for purposes of Medicaid eligibility, it is your net equity that counts. In other words, an asset's value is the price that it can reasonably be expected to sell for on the open market in the particular geographic area involved, minus any encumbrances (i.e., debt) on the asset. Note that if you have $10,000 in cash in the bank, and $10,000 in credit card debt, the debt will *not* be netted against the cash! You will need to pay off the debt, otherwise Medicaid will simply count that $10,000 toward your asset limit, ignoring the debt.

Countable Assets

If you can spend it or convert it to cash, it is generally countable. Here are the primary examples of "countable" assets:

- Cash, checking and savings accounts
- CDs
- Stocks, bonds, mutual funds
- IRA, 401(k), 403(b), TIAA-CREF, and other retirement-type accounts (with exceptions discussed below)

- Life insurance cash values (if the total face value of all policies exceeds $1,500)
- Annuities not yet in pay status
- All autos beyond the first car
- Trucks, tractors, boats, machinery, livestock
- Buildings and land that is not specifically excluded

Unavailable Assets

Certain types of assets are non-countable, because they are not legally accessible to you:

- an interest in someone's estate, prior to distribution
- a lawsuit you've filed, prior to the judgment
- real estate that cannot be sold because of legal technicalities

Excluded Assets

Certain assets, while still available and accessible to you, are nonetheless considered "excluded" or "exempt," i.e., they will not affect your eligibility for Medicaid.

$2,000 Cash

Regardless of whether you are single or married, if you are successful in qualifying for Medicaid coverage you may retain up to $2,000 in cash or other countable assets. In any month where your assets exceed $2,000, however, you could be disqualified and lose Medicaid coverage. Since that would cause you to lose all nursing home and medical coverage, that would be a very expensive mistake. Accordingly, be careful always to keep the bank account of the Medicaid recipient well below the $2,000 limit!

The Home

GENERAL RULE: $500,000 EXCLUSION. If you are single, and your principal place of residence is a house or condo, it is an excluded asset, so long as your equity interest in the residence does not exceed the state limit (at least

$500,000, but this amount can be increased up to $750,000 under federal law, *if* the state you are in so chooses; most have not done so). The home *used to be* excluded no matter its value, but that changed with the DRA of 2005, effective 1/1/06 (note this date, which is earlier than the effective date of 2/8/06 for most other DRA provisions).

Note that it is the value of your *equity interest*, not the value of the home itself that is critical. In other words, if you and your brother are equal joint owners of the house you live in, and the home has been appraised at $800,000, your equity interest is only one-half of that, i.e., $400,000, so you are under the limit. Of course, if you were the *sole* owner, then you'd be over the limit.

If the value of your equity interest in your home is above the state limit, in order for the home to be excluded you will need to reduce your equity interest. How can you do that? This is covered on page 82.

If the value of your equity interest in your home is under the state limit when you first apply for Medicaid, the home will be an excluded asset. But be aware that if the value of your home has increased above the state limit at the time of your annual redetermination, the home will no longer be excluded and you can lose your Medicaid coverage! Thus, it is extremely important for your family to keep track of the value of your home, and if it looks like it's getting over the state limit, you'll need to implement one of the options discussed on page 82, to reduce your equity interest.

If you are married and your spouse resides in the home, or you have a child (under age 21, or blind or permanently disabled) living in your home, then it is excluded no matter what its value is.

SCOPE OF THE EXCLUSION. Both the dwelling *and* the land underneath it qualify for the home exclusion. You do not need to own the dwelling: you can be living in someone else's trailer on your land, and the land will be excluded under the home exclusion.

The home itself, the land the home sits on, all contiguous land, and related outbuildings are all covered by the exclusion. (If the adjoining lot is across the street from your house, it still qualifies as being contiguous.) So a house and attached farm can all be excluded. Of course, there is still the

$500,000 exclusion limitation (unless one of the exceptions applies: spouse or child—under age 21, or blind or permanently disabled—living in the home).

A mobile home or a houseboat both qualify for the home exclusion.

"INTENT TO RETURN." If you have to move out of your home and into a nursing home, the home will continue to be an excluded asset under the rules discussed above, with the same limitations, *if* you have *the intent to return* to your home should you ever become well enough to leave the nursing home. This rule applies no matter how unlikely it is that you'll ever recover to the point where you are able to leave the nursing home. If you are incapacitated to the point where you are unable to communicate your intent to return home, a spouse or dependent relative is permitted to express your intent on your behalf. However, to be on the safe side, it is a good idea for you—as soon as you move out of your home into a nursing home—to sign a statement explicitly stating that if you are ever well enough, your intent is to return to residing in your old home. This can be useful to show to the Medicaid authorities should it become necessary to document your intent to return.

What if you leave your home of many years and move to an assisted living facility and then later into a nursing home? Will the former home still be excluded? No, since the former home is no longer your principal place of residence. Obviously, a short hospital stay in between the transition from your home to a nursing home will not cause you to lose the home exclusion. But any reasonable time where you moved your permanent residence from your old home to a new home, apartment, or assisted living facility, could certainly prevent your former home from being an excluded asset. The key test is if you continued to "intend to return" to your former home. For example, the regulations of some states provide that the home will no longer be excluded if you moved out more than six months before you entered the nursing home. Of course, if your spouse or child (under age 21, or blind or permanently disabled) remains in your old home, it will continue to be excluded regardless of whether you go directly from that home to a nursing home.

SALE OF THE HOME. If you or your spouse sells the home, the proceeds from the sale will continue to be excluded so long as they are reinvested in another excluded home within three months of the sale. Whatever is not reinvested will become countable. Thus, if you are single, those extra proceeds could cause you to lose your Medicaid eligibility. If you are married and on Medicaid, the extra proceeds may be safely retained by the Community Spouse and will not cause you (the nursing home spouse) to become ineligible for Medicaid.

> That's because of the federal statute that states that the assets of the Community Spouse cannot be deemed available to the nursing home spouse starting with the month after the month in which the nursing home spouse is declared eligible for Medicaid coverage.

One Automobile

One automobile of any value is excluded. Until recently, an auto was only excluded up to $4,500 in value, but that limitation is now gone. Once you go past that first car, additional vehicles will be countable assets, at their fair market value (less any outstanding car loan). See *New Auto, Bigger Auto*, page 77, for some planning ideas related to cars.

Personal Property

Under the federal regulations as amended on March 9, 2005, all household goods (furniture, furnishings, TV, computer, etc.) and personal effects (jewelry, clothing, etc.) are now excluded when determining a person's Medicaid eligibility. This is so regardless of their value. "Household goods" must be items of personal property found in or near a home, that are used on a regular basis, or items needed by the householder for maintenance, use and occupancy of the premises as a home. "Personal effects" are considered items of personal property that ordinarily are worn or carried by the individual, or are articles that otherwise have an intimate relation to the individual. Items with religious or cultural significance are also excluded under these rules. Items held for investment purposes, though, are *not* excluded and their value will be counted: items such as gems, jewelry that is not worn or held for family significance, recently purchased expensive artwork, and other collectibles.

How will the Medicaid workers know whether your household goods, furniture, etc., are normal household items, or if such items are really "held for investment" or "collectibles"? According to the federal regulations, "we will not routinely examine all of an individual's furniture and personal possessions to determine if any pieces are valuable artwork or antiques, [but] we will have the regulatory authority to count such value items as resources when we become aware of such items."

While it is true that your wedding ring and other personal jewelry are excluded, do not run out and purchase expensive jewelry and expect it to be excluded. This was tried in a famous Massachusetts case, where the individual in question, in an attempt to qualify for Medicaid, purchased a $45,000 diamond ring. Unfortunately, the judge ruled that this jewelry item was not excluded but was a countable investment asset. So the moral of the story is, don't get greedy!

Funeral and Burial Funds

BANK ACCOUNT. Up to $1,500 may be placed in a bank account, revocable account, trust or other arrangement, and if it is designated as a burial fund, it will be excluded from your countable assets. However, this exclusion must be reduced by (i) the amount of any irrevocable burial funds such as that described in the next section, and (ii) the face value of any life insurance policy whose cash value is excluded (see *Life Insurance*, page 41). For a married couple, the $1,500 exclusion applies to each spouse.

PRE-PAID FUNERAL/BURIAL. There is no practical limit to the amount you can set aside in a pre-paid burial and funeral account established with a funeral home or in an irrevocable trust earmarked only for payment of your funeral and burial expenses. With a funeral home, the money must either be placed in an escrow account or trust account by the funeral home. Some states require that the contract specifically state that any funds in the account not ultimately used for funeral and burial expenses following your death must be paid to the state if you were on Medicaid. In any event, you should not put more into such an account than you believe you will actually need to pay for these expenses; having any sort of pre-arranged "deal" with the funeral home to pay the excess to your family is clearly illegal.

LIFE INSURANCE. Life insurance earmarked for burial expenses ("burial insurance"), where the proceeds can only be used for burial expenses, is an excluded asset.

FAMILY COVERAGE. Not only can you pre-pay funeral and burial expenses for yourself (and your spouse, if any), but you are also permitted to prepay the burial space costs for the following family members: your children (of any age), stepchildren, adopted children, brothers, sisters, parents, adoptive parents, and the spouses of any of those persons. This includes burial plots, gravesites, crypts, mausoleums, urns, niches, and other customary and traditional repositories for the deceased's remains, provided such spaces are owned by the individual. It also includes vaults, headstones, markers, plaques, and burial containers, and arrangements for opening and closing the gravesite for the burial.

IRAs

If the Medicaid applicant is unmarried, then the IRA or other retirement asset (such as 401(k), 403(b), etc.) is countable, the same as cash. Some states recognize that if the retirement assets were withdrawn to pay bills, there would be a substantial income tax due on the withdrawn amount. Accordingly, those states will reduce the "countable" amount by an estimated amount of the tax, e.g., 20%. If no such reduction is permitted in your state, you may be better off withdrawing the entire amount of the retirement assets and paying the taxes immediately as an estimated tax, since otherwise Medicaid will ignore the amount of taxes you *will* owe on that withdrawal come next year once you file your income tax return, in effect over-valuing your retirement assets by the amount of the tax you'll owe. If the withdrawal will kick you into a higher tax bracket, try to withdraw half this year and half on January 2 of next year; that will divide the taxable distributions between two tax years, possibly saving you some money.

If the Medicaid applicant is married, many states do not count the retirement assets of the Community Spouse. In these states, then, the Community Spouse may retain the $101,640 CSRA (see page 42) in addition to any retirement assets. Other states are not so generous and count the retirement assets of both spouses the same as cash in the bank.

Property Used in a Trade or Business

According to federal law, real or personal property "essential to self-support" that is currently used in a trade or business is excluded from resources *regardless of its value* or rate of return.

For example, if you have a working farm, the land, tool sheds, livestock and equipment would all be excluded. A small family-owned business would also qualify under this exclusion. This seems to have little application to an unmarried individual who is in a nursing home, since such person will of course not be able to argue that he or she is currently using such property for self-support. However, for a married couple, it could exclude a significant amount of property so long as it is still in current use by the Community Spouse in a trade or business or as an employee. Unfortunately, many states have ignored this rule or limited it to the $6,000/6% amount discussed below, which should only be applied to *non*-business property.

Non-Business Property Used for Self-Support

If real or personal property is *not* used in a trade or business, only the first $6,000 of value is excluded, *if* it generates at least a 6% return on the amount excluded.

Example:

If you own a separate lot of land worth $10,000, and you rent it out to someone who moved his own mobile home onto the lot, as long as it generates at least $600 of income each year, $6,000 of the land's value may be excluded (the income must be prorated to the entire lot).

Life Insurance

Only the cash value of a life insurance policy owned by the Medicaid applicant is counted; thus, all term life insurance policies are ignored. Also, if the total face value of all life insurance policies is less than $1,500, then the cash value is ignored.

If you are applying for Medicaid and already have a term policy in effect, you won't be able to divert any of your income to keep that policy in force, once you are on Medicaid. If your family realizes that your life expectancy is reduced and thus it makes sense not to let the policy lapse, they should consider paying the annual premiums themselves, out of their own pockets. It is also advisable to transfer ownership of the policy to another family member, so they will be the one to receive premium notices, etc.

Married

Community Spouse Resource Allowance (CSRA)

The basic rules discussed above as to when an asset is counted, unavailable or excluded apply to married couples and unmarried individuals alike. In either case, the person applying for Medicaid cannot have more than $2,000 in countable assets. The big difference is that under the Medicaid rules the Community Spouse is allowed to own a certain amount of assets (i.e., resources) that do not count against the $2,000 that the nursing home spouse is permitted to own. This *"protected amount" is known as the Community Spouse Resource Allowance, or CSRA.* All other countable assets owned by the couple, regardless of which spouse owns the asset, must be "spent down," converted into non-countable assets, or otherwise disposed of by the couple, before the nursing home spouse will be eligible for Medicaid.

NOTE: If *both* spouses are in the nursing home and applying for Medicaid, then there is no CSRA (because there is no Community Spouse) and the total countable assets of both spouses cannot exceed $3,000.

Let's take a look at how the CSRA is determined.

"Snapshot" Rule

Regardless of whether a married nursing home resident applies for Medicaid immediately upon entering the nursing home or some months later, the CSRA is based on the value of the couple's assets as of the date the nursing home spouse first entered the nursing home. To be precise, this "snapshot" is taken on the first day of the month in which the nursing home spouse is in the nursing home (or a patient in the hospital just prior to entering the nursing home, as the case may be) and likely to remain there for a continuous period of at least 30 consecutive days.

Unlike how *income* is separately counted for each spouse, a married couple's *assets* are simply added together when determining the allowable assets each spouse can keep. Thus, it doesn't matter how an asset is titled: husband's name, wife's name, or joint names—it's all treated the same for these purposes. (Note that community property rules and pre-nuptial and post-nuptial agreements are all ignored for purposes of calculating the CSRA.)

As a practical matter, when one spouse of a married couple is in a nursing home and it appears that Medicaid assistance may be needed at some point, the Community Spouse should make an appointment with a caseworker at the local office of the state department of human services to request a "resource assessment." This is *not* the same as applying for Medicaid, which as a general rule *should not be done* until it is *certain* that the spouse will indeed qualify at such time. (For the consequences of applying for Medicaid too early, see page 16.) The "resource assessment" will establish the total value of a married couple's countable

assets as of the "snapshot" date, for purposes of calculating the CSRA. The longer the couple waits to apply for Medicaid, the more difficult it can be to recreate the assets owned by the couple on the "snapshot" date as well as what the assets were worth at that time. Hence, it is always better to get the resource assessment done as soon as possible after a spouse enters the nursing home.

Once the total countable assets as of the snapshot date are determined, the Community Spouse is allowed to keep a portion of those assets (i.e., the CSRA). The CSRA calculation varies from state to state, as discussed below.

Fifty Percent States

In some states, the Community Spouse may protect no more than 50% of the total countable assets of the couple, with a minimum CSRA of $20,328 and a maximum CSRA of $101,640 (federal figures, updated annually). Some of these states round up the minimum figure to, for example, $25,000.

Example 1:

Joe (at home) and Mary (in the nursing home) have a total of $21,000 in countable assets. Joe can keep the greater of $20,328 or 50% of their combined assets. Since 50% of $21,000 is less than $20,328, Joe gets to keep $20,328, and Mary can keep the balance of their assets— $672. Since Mary has less than $2,000, she can immediately apply for Medicaid without having to spend down any of the couple's assets.

Example 2:

What if Joe and Mary had $150,000? You start by taking 50% of that amount, which is $75,000. Since that's more than $20,328 but less than the maximum permitted amount of $101,640, Joe can keep that $75,000, while Mary is deemed the owner of the other half, i.e., $75,000. Since Mary is only permitted to have $2,000, she would not qualify for Medicaid until her excess assets—$73,000—were disposed of in some way.

Example 3:

What if Joe and Mary had $250,000, instead? Once again, you start by taking 50% of that amount, which is $125,000. But since that exceeds $101,640, Joe is only permitted to protect $101,640. The balance— $148,360—is deemed to be Mary's. Since Mary is only permitted to have $2,000, she would not qualify for Medicaid until her excess assets—$146,360—were disposed of in some way.

NOTE: If you reside in a "fifty percent state," and the total countable assets of you and your spouse are between $20,328 and $101,640, there is a way where you can *increase* the amount of your countable assets and thereby increase the CSRA. This must be done before one spouse enters the nursing home, because it must be completed before the "snapshot" date. This is explained in detail in *Converting Non-Countable Assets to Countable* (page 79).

Hundred Percent States

In the other states, the Community Spouse may keep 100% of the total countable assets of the couple, *up to* the maximum amount (currently $101,640). There is no "minimum" CSRA in these states.

Example 1:

Joe (at home) and Mary (in the nursing home) have a total of $21,000. Joe can keep all of the assets, since they're less than $101,640.

Example 2:

Joe and Mary have a total of $80,000. Joe keeps not just $40,000, but the full $80,000, since that's less than $101,640.

Example 3:

If Joe and Mary had $150,000, Joe keeps the first $101,640, and Mary is considered the owner of the balance—$48,360. Since Mary is only permitted to have $2,000, she would not qualify for Medicaid until her excess assets—$46,360—were disposed of in some way.

Increasing the CSRA

Up until now, we have been looking at ways of calculating the default CSRA. If the couple is not satisfied with the state determination of the CSRA, it may be possible to get an increase. There are two ways to do this: apply for a Fair Hearing or obtain a court order of support for the Community Spouse.

Fair Hearing

A Fair Hearing is an administrative appeal within the Medicaid state agency that makes the determination of financial eligibility for Medicaid. It is usually an informal proceeding, but it is a good idea to bring an attorney with you if possible.

Since the DRA's effective date of February 8, 2006, all states must now use the "income first" approach in setting the CSRA. That means that if the Community Spouse's income can be brought up to the MMMNA level by shifting income from the nursing home spouse, then the CSRA may not be increased. However, if the income of *both* spouses is *still* under the MMMNA, then it is possible to request an increase in the CSRA by an amount of assets sufficient to generate the additional income needed to bring the Community Spouse up to the MMMNA level.

Example:

Bart is in the nursing home and his only income is $500/month of Social Security. His wife, Louise, lives in the community and her only income is $1,000/month of Social Security. Under the MMMNA rules discussed above, because Louise's income is less than $1,650/month, Louise will be allowed to keep all of Bart's income. However, that still leaves her short $150/month ($1,650 − 1,000 - $500 = $150).

Because of this, Louise will be entitled to keep an additional amount of the couple's assets, based on the reasoning that those additional assets will be needed to generate that additional $150/month of income. It works like this: if Louise can only expect typically to earn 5% on her money, then it will take what amount of additional assets to generate that $150/month shortfall? The formula is:

5% of x = $150 month or $1,800/yr; so x = $1,800 ÷ 5% = $36,000.

Result:

Louise can protect not just the CSRA of $101,640, but an *additional* $36,000 of the couple's assets. Once they have reduced their assets to that level, Bart can apply for Medicaid.

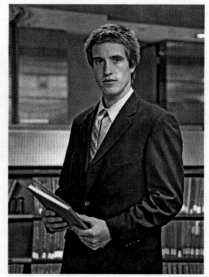

Note that the 5% income figure used above is merely an example. Some states set the percentage you must use; others let you argue at the Fair Hearing what an appropriate percent should be, based on an average of local CD rates, etc. Other states require you to obtain estimates of the cost of a single premium lifetime annuity sufficient to generate the income shortfall, and the average of the estimated costs of that annuity is the amount by which you can increase the CSRA (you don't actually have to *buy* the annuity, however). Thus, the particular rules of your state must be consulted before you go into the Fair Hearing.

Here's where it pays to work hard for an increased MMMNA (see page 29 about how to do this). If Mary were able to increase her MMMNA from the default minimum of $1,650 to the maximum of $2,541, that additional $891/ month allowed income would permit her to protect an additional $213,840 of assets as part of her CSRA! Here's how the numbers work:

Maximum MMMNA	$2,541
Default MMMNA	(1,650)
Increase/month	891
Increase/year	10,692
Amount of assets required to generate $10,692/yr, at 5% interest	$213,840

Court Orders

If the Community Spouse finds that he or she simply cannot make ends meet with the default minimum amounts of income or assets allowed under the Medicaid rules, the Community Spouse should seek a Court Order of Support to increase either or both of these amounts. If an Order is obtained to increase the spouse's allowed income (i.e., the MMMNA), then the next step is to request a Fair Hearing to shift additional assets under the analysis discussed above. It is also possible to obtain a Court Order to increase the CSRA itself. These Orders must be recognized by the Medicaid agency in determining the amount of income or assets the Community Spouse is entitled to keep, while still allowing the nursing home spouse to qualify for Medicaid. The petition to the Court should be done prior to applying for Medicaid, but may be done before or after the "resource assessment."

A Court Order may also be sought if additional assets (CSRA) are needed for the support of a "family member" (minor or dependent children, dependent parents, or dependent siblings of the nursing home spouse or of the Community Spouse who are residing with the Community Spouse). For example, an elderly parent or sibling may be residing with the Community

Spouse; as a result, a Court Order of support can increase the assets available to cover the costs associated with supporting that family member through a higher CSRA.

Post-Eligibility Increases to the CSRA

Under the federal statute, after the month in which the nursing home spouse is initially determined to be eligible for Medicaid "no resources of the community spouse shall be deemed available to the institutionalized spouse." That's exactly how the Court held in a 2004 U.S. Court of Appeals case. Thus, even if the Community Spouse's assets double in value because of good investment performance—or if the Community Spouse wins the lottery or receives an inheritance—those additional assets will not affect the nursing home spouse's Medicaid eligibility and need not be contributed toward the nursing home spouse's care. Although annual redeterminations must be made of the nursing home spouse's assets and income, no such annual redeterminations are necessary or permitted of the Community Spouse's assets.

Chapter 8

TRANSFERRING ASSETS (GIFTS)

Penalty Period

If you make a gift to anyone other than your spouse, you will be ineligible to receive Medicaid assistance for a certain period of time known as the "penalty" period. During this period, even if your assets and income are within the range that would normally allow you to qualify for Medicaid, so long as you are within the penalty period you will be denied Medicaid coverage, barring a hardship exception.

The length of this "penalty period" depends on the value of your gift. The larger the gift, the longer the penalty period. You calculate this penalty period by taking the value of the gifted assets and dividing that value by the average cost of a nursing home in your state. (Every state publishes this "divisor" figure and typically updates it annually, to adjust for inflation.)

It makes no difference how many recipients of the gifts there are. Whether the gift is made to one person or ten, the penalty period is figured the same way: it is based on the total amount of all gifts made during the lookback period. (Do not confuse this rule with the federal law that exempts $12,000 per gift recipient per year. So for gift tax purposes it does indeed matter whether the gift is made to one person or ten—but not for Medicaid purposes!)

If you are married, the same penalty period applies whether the gift is made by the person who will be applying for Medicaid or that person's spouse. So having your spouse make the gift instead of you makes no difference.

Example:

Let's assume the divisor figure in your state—as determined by your Medicaid department—is $5,000 per month. So if you wrote a check to your daughter for $50,000, you would be ineligible for Medicaid assistance for 10 months: $50,000 gift divided by $5,000 divisor = 10 months.

Now this next point is critical: **There is no limit on the length of the penalty period.**

For example, if you deeded your $350,000 house to your daughter and son today, and if your state divisor figure were \$5,000, the penalty period would be 70 months: \$350,000 divided by \$5,000 = 70 months. I hear you say, "But I thought there is a five-year limit on the penalty?" Five years refers to the "lookback period" (discussed in the next section), not the penalty period. It is important not to confuse the two concepts. Therefore, you could avoid the 70-month penalty simply by not applying for Medicaid until after the 60th month, at which point the gift will be outside the lookback period. So if you applied for Medicaid in month 61, the gift of the house is ignored, so you would immediately be eligible. Let me give you another example.

Example:

On March 1, 2006, John transfers his \$250,000 house and \$50,000 in cash to his three children. How long must he wait to be eligible for Medicaid benefits? Assuming the state divisor figure is \$5,000, John will be ineligible for Medicaid for 60 months, or five years: total amount of gifts (\$250,000 + \$50,000 = \$300,000) divided by \$5,000 = 60 months. So if John applied for Medicaid on March 1, 2007, before the lookback period had expired, he would be told he was ineligible for Medicaid for another five years, i.e., until March 1, 2012. Clearly he would be better off not to apply until *at least* after March 1, 2011; at that point, the gifts will be ignored since they would be outside of the lookback period. Result: an extra year of Medicaid coverage, saving his family \$60,000-\$80,000 or more.

NOTE: Be sure to check with an experienced elder law attorney in your state if you are about to apply for Medicaid after a lookback period. Different states calculate this differently, and it's better to apply slightly too late than a day too early!

Penalty Start Date: Pre-DRA Gifts

As to any gift made before February 8, 2006, the penalty start date in most states is the first day of the month in which the gift is made (some states start with the following month). In other words, if you wrote a check to your daughter on January 20, 2006, you would normally calculate the penalty period as if you had made the gift on January 1, 2006.

Penalty Start Date: Post-DRA Gifts

As to any gift made on or after February 8, 2006, the penalty start date is the date on which the Medicaid applicant would have been eligible to receive Medicaid coverage but for the imposition of the gift penalty, or, if later, the first day of the month in which the gift is made.

NOTE: The state will use the divisor in effect at the time you apply for Medicaid, not the one in effect on the date of the gift. For example, if you make a gift of $50,000 today when the divisor is $5,000, but you apply for Medicaid four years from now, when the divisor has been increased to $5,500, the penalty will be only 9.1 months, not 10 months.

Tacking

What if you make a gift while a penalty period is still running, from an earlier gift you made? For pre-DRA gifts (i.e., made before 2/8/06), the additional gift is "tacked on" to the end of the existing penalty period. For post-DRA gifts (i.e., made on or after 2/8/06), all gifts made within the lookback period are simply added together, and the number of months penalty period is based on the total of all those gifts.

Example of Pre-DRA Gifts (made before 2/8/06):

On January 1, 2005, you made a $100,000 gift. Assuming the divisor is $5,000, that causes a penalty of 20 months, i.e., until September 1, 2006. If you made a second gift of, say, $10,000, on August 15, 2005, you would simply tack on an additional two months ($10,000 / $5,000) to the end of the prior penalty period. So you would be ineligible for Medicaid until November 1, 2006.

Post-DRA Gifts (made on or after 2/8/06):

On March 1, 2006, you made a gift of $10,000, on May 1, 2007, you made a gift of $15,000, and on April 1, 2009, you made a gift of $20,000. On July 1, 2010, you applied for Medicaid. Since all these gifts were made within the lookback period (i.e., within five years preceding the date you applied for Medicaid), you would face a penalty period based on the total amount of gifts made within this period ($45,000), and the penalty period would start running as of the date you applied for Medicaid. If the state divisor were $5,000, then the penalty period would be nine months, i.e., until April 1, 2011.

Valuing the Gift

The general rule is that the value of a gifted asset is its "fair market value." That means what you could sell it for in a retail sale to the general public in a private party sale.

Automobiles

Look up the Kelly Blue Book value (www.kbb.com). Remember, however, that the one auto is excluded no matter what its value is.

Bank Accounts, CDs

Value is based on the amount you would receive if you liquidated the account. So for a CD, only count the amount of interest already credited to your account.

Life Insurance

Only cash value is counted, so ignore the value of term insurance, which has no cash value. Contact the insurance company to obtain a Form 712, which will set forth the current cash value less outstanding loans, if any. That will be the value for Medicaid purposes.

Real Estate

For real estate, you may need to get an appraisal, although often you can rely on the 100% value as stated on your most recent real estate tax bill. This is usually spelled out in your state Medicaid regulations.

Stocks, Bonds, Mutual Funds

Since the values of these assets fluctuate daily, obtain the value as of the date of the gift.

Partial Gifts

Occasionally people get the bright idea that if they "sell" some item they own to their children for, say, a dollar, then the entire transaction is no longer a gift. After all, it was a sale, not a gift, right? Unfortunately, that technique doesn't work. In reality, this transaction will be characterized as a part gift/part sale. The amount of compensation received will be subtracted from the fair market value of the asset that was transferred, to arrive at the value of the gift. So if you sell your house to your daughter for $10,000, and the house was appraised at $200,000, then you have made a gift of $190,000 ($200,000 - $10,000).

Lookback Period

When a person applies for Medicaid, one of the questions on the intake form will be "Have you (or your spouse, if married) made any gifts within the past 60 months?" (Note that a gift by your spouse counts the same as a gift by you.) What the Medicaid workers are looking for are "uncompensated transfers" or "transfers without fair consideration," i.e., gifts, so that they can impose the proper penalty period (discussed above). If the gift was made too long ago, it must be ignored; it would be as if you never made the gift at all, no matter how large a gift it was. How far back the worker can look to see if you made a gift is known as the "lookback period." There are several considerations that apply to gifts, depending on whether they were made "pre-DRA" (i.e., before 2/8/06) or "post-DRA: (i.e., on or after 2/8/06) and if they were outright (i.e., given directly to an individual) or made to a trust.

Outright Gifts

When the penalty for gifting was first implemented, the lookback period for outright gifts was 24 months. It was later extended to 30 months, then 36 months and finally to the current period of 60 months. This means that any gift you made more than 60 months prior to the date you apply for Medicaid must be ignored. For example, if you transfer your million dollar house to your children but do not apply for Medicaid until 61 months later, then this very large gift must be ignored and will not count against you.

Under the rules effective for post-DRA gifts, there is no benefit to making a gift sooner rather than later unless the person who makes the gift can wait at least a full *five years* from the date of the gift. That is because the penalty period does not begin to run until the person who made the gift applies for Medicaid.

Example:

Sally has only $102,000 of countable assets. Thinking she may need to move into a nursing home in a couple of years, Sally makes a gift of $50,000 on January 1 of next year (Year 1) and another $50,000 on January 1 of the year after that (Year 2). On January 1 of Year 4, Sally has to move into a nursing home. By this time she has no countable assets left (other than her personal exclusion of $2,000), so ordinarily she would have qualified for Medicaid. However, since she made gifts within the past five years of her application date, the two $50,000 gifts must be added together and treated as if she made the gifts on the day she applied for Medicaid. So her $100,000 of total gifts will now cause her to be disqualified for a period equal to $100,000 ÷ $5,000 [assuming that's the state penalty divisor figure] = 20 months. If Sally waits until January 1 of Year 6, only the second gift of $50,000 will count against her, since the first gift is now more than 5 years old. Finally, if Sally instead waits until January 1 of year 7, then she will immediately qualify for Medicaid, because more than 5 years have passed since the date of her last gift.

DRA Transition Rules

Outright gifts made on or after February 8, 2006, are subject to the new 60-month lookback rule. Since the old rule still applies as to any gifts made *prior* to this date, this change really will have no effect until more than three years have gone by, i.e., after February 8, 2009. At that point, the lookback period as to outright gifts will be extended one month for each month that passes. In other words, for an application made on December 8, 2009, the lookback period for outright gifts will be three years, 10 months (i.e., only back to February 8, 2006), and *not* 60 months. The Medicaid workers cannot go back further than that, because any gifts made before February 8, 2006, were only subject to a 36-month lookback period, and we're already beyond that at this point in time.

Gifts to Trusts

Different rules apply to gifts into and out of revocable and irrevocable trusts. See the discussion in Chapter 9, *Trusts*.

Taxable Gifts

If you live in Connecticut, Louisiana, North Carolina, or Tennessee, there is a state gift tax, independent of the federal gift tax. The federal gift tax will rarely be an issue, since it exempts the first $1,000,000 of lifetime gifts. Although Connecticut has an even higher lifetime exemption ($2,000,000), the other three have much lower thresholds: Tennessee ($12,000 annual exclusion for gifts to children; no separate lifetime exemption); Louisiana ($30,000); North Carolina ($100,000). These amounts apply to gifts that are made to children in excess of $12,000 per year per child.

Example:

Bobby Lee deeds her Tennessee house to her son, when it is valued at $250,000. Under Tennessee law, she will owe the state gift taxes of $15,070 on this transfer.

Chapter 9

TRUSTS

Basic Terms and Concepts

> A "trust" is a legal arrangement where one person (called the "trustee") holds and manages property for the benefit of someone else (the "beneficiary"). The terms of the trust document control what the trustee may do with the trust property. It will set forth specific instructions for how the property can be invested as well as who can receive distributions from the trust and under what circumstances.

Trust "property" can be any type of asset that can be titled in the name of a trust, such as cash, CDs, stocks, or real estate. The property in the trust is called the "principal" of the trust. Any interest, dividends or other income generated by the trust property is called the trust "income."

You can actually wear more than one hat: you can be the creator of the trust (called the "grantor" or "settlor" of the trust), the trustee, *and* the beneficiary!

There are two basic types of trusts—revocable and irrevocable—and the Medicaid rules that apply to trusts differ depending on which type you create. Let's take a look at these two types of trusts.

Revocable Trusts

> A "revocable" trust is one that can be changed or revoked by the creator of the trust, at any time. A revocable trust is what is commonly referred to as a "Living Trust." Such trusts are widely promoted in seminars as offering a tremendous number of benefits over a will. However, as a general rule, revocable trusts are not recommended for Medicaid planning purposes.

All Trust Assets Countable

If a Medicaid applicant (or spouse) has the power to revoke a trust, then *all* the assets titled in the name of that trust will be countable for purposes of determining the eligibility of the applicant. For example, if you transferred your car into the name of the trust, the car, which is normally excluded if owned in your own name, would now be countable. This applies to your home, too. Although your home is normally an excluded asset, if the home is deeded into the name of your revocable trust, it loses its exclusion and will now be a countable asset! If this is your situation, you will need to deed the house out of the trust name and put it back into your name (or your spouse's name, if you are married) before you apply for Medicaid. (For the one exception, see *Converting Non-Countable Assets to Countable*, page 79.)

Transfers To and From

There is never a penalty for transferring assets from your name into the name of your revocable trust. But should you make a distribution from the trust to a beneficiary of the trust, it's treated the same as if you made a gift of those same assets yourself, directly, i.e., in most cases subject to a penalty (see page 50) and the five-year lookback period (see page 54).

Revocable trusts can be great for estate planning purposes, by avoiding probate, permitting a consolidated management of your assets in the event you become disabled, ensuring privacy of your estate plan, etc. But they are rarely used for Medicaid planning purposes for an *unmarried* individual, for the reasons discussed above. Be careful if anyone suggests to you that a "Living Trust" can protect you from Medicaid claims and hasten your eligibility—remember that all assets titled in the name of a Living Trust are countable assets for purposes of Medicaid eligibility.

On the other hand, there can be *some* benefit for a married Medicaid applicant, if the Community Spouse can transfer all of the Community Spouse's assets into a revocable trust and—in some states— eliminate the right of the nursing home spouse to force a distribution from the estate of the Community Spouse should the Community Spouse predecease the nursing home spouse. This will be discussed in greater detail below.

Irrevocable Trusts

An "irrevocable" trust is one that cannot be changed or revoked by the creator of the trust. Irrevocable trusts can be very useful for Medicaid planning purposes.

Transfers To and From

If you transfer an asset into the name of an irrevocable trust, is it considered a gift? The test is whether any portion of the trust may be distributed back to you for any reason under any circumstances. If so, then that portion of the trust is treated as an available asset to you, i.e., the same as if you had put the asset into a revocable trust. If there are *no* circumstances in which the assets you put into the trust can be distributed back to you, then your transferring those assets into the trust is a gift. This would be calculated the same way as a gift to an individual. For example, if you transfer $100,000 into the name of an irrevocable trust and the terms of the trust state that only $10,000 can ever be distributed back to you *if* you had serious medical problems, then (i) $10,000 (i.e., 10%) of the trust is counted as an available asset to you for Medicaid purposes, and (ii) the balance of $90,000 is deemed a gift from you, subject to a penalty and the five-year lookback period.

If the trust states that distributions may be made back to you but also may be made to someone *other than you*, such as your children, then any distribution out of the trust to this other beneficiary is deemed a gift *from* you (and therefore subject to a penalty and the five-year lookback period— although a gift *out* of such a trust that was made before 2/8/06 is only subject to a *three*-year lookback period).

If the trust does not permit distributions of principal back to you under any circumstances, then your transfer of assets to such a trust is a gift, as explained above. In addition, any distributions from such a trust *to someone other than you* are ignored, because the penalty was imposed when you initially transferred the property *into* the trust. They can't penalize you twice for transferring the same property!

If the trust states that the income *or* the principal of the trust can be distributed back to you, any distribution from the trust to you is treated as income to you (for Medicaid purposes; different rules apply for income tax purposes).

If income *can* be distributed to you, in the trustee's discretion, but is withheld for any reason, that income is treated as a resource of yours. If you are already covered by Medicaid, be sure that any such income does not accumulate, possibly putting you over the $2,000 limit. The way to avoid that is for the trust to distribute all such income to you (or to your spouse, if any) so it does not accumulate.

Planning with Irrevocable Trusts

Once your transfer to the trust is considered a gift, it is no longer a countable asset of yours. That is why irrevocable trusts can be excellent long-term planning vehicles: Once the lookback period has expired, the trust is ignored. So if you transfer all your assets into the right kind of irrevocable trust and wait out the five-year lookback period, the assets in the name of the trust, no matter their value, will not count against you when you apply for Medicaid. (See *Lookback Period*, page 54.)

Example:

Assume you are age 65 and believe that you are in pretty good health with little likelihood of needing nursing home care for many years. However, you are concerned that if you did have to go to a nursing home someday, the costs would deplete your estate. Instead, you'd like to leave your estate to your children, if at all possible. Accordingly, you go to your elder law attorney to draw up an irrevocable trust, and you transfer $300,000 (or a parcel of real estate—even your home) into the trust.

After five years have passed from the date you transferred the money or property into the trust, that transfer will be outside the five-year lookback period and thus cannot count against you. You can even serve as trustee of your own trust, so you will continue to manage and control the trust assets for the rest of your life. You can include a provision allowing discretionary distributions to your children and grandchildren out of the trust, giving you the power to make gifts to them at any time in any amount. If it is your home that you put into the trust, you can reserve the right to live in the house for the rest of your life. You, as trustee, can sell the house and purchase another house, or a condo, and if there are extra proceeds from the sale of the house, they would remain as part of the trust, protected from Medicaid claims.

Example 1:

Joe transfers $100,000 into a revocable "living" trust. He withdraws $5,000 a month later to pay some bills, and a month after that he writes a $20,000 check from the trust to his daughter, to help her with a down payment on a house.

RESULT: There is no penalty period imposed upon Joe's initial transfer of $100,000 into the trust, because he can revoke the trust at any time and get it all back. Also, should he apply for Medicaid, all of the assets in the trust will be countable as his own money, just as if he had not placed them in the name of the trust. This is true regardless of when he established the trust.

The gift to his daughter will be a disqualifying transfer subject to a 60-month lookback period. That means that if Joe applies for Medicaid within 60 months from the date he wrote the check, then assuming the state penalty divisor is $5,000, such gift will cause a four-month penalty period. If he wrote her the check prior to February 8, 2006, the penalty period started to run on the date he gave her the check so it has already expired. If he gave her the check on or after February 8, 2006, the penalty will run from the day he applies for Medicaid.

Example 2:

Continuing the above Example 1, a year later—when the trust is worth $80,000—Joe decides to make his revocable trust irrevocable, but he retains the right to the income, only. In no circumstance, however, may the trustee distribute any of the underlying trust principal to him. On the date he makes the trust irrevocable, he is treated as having made a gift of $80,000 to the other trust beneficiaries. Should Joe apply for Medicaid within 60 months of that date, he will be faced with a penalty period of $80,000 divided by the state penalty period divisor. So if the divisor is $5,000, then the penalty period will be 16 months. Again, the penalty will not start to run until the day he applies for Medicaid.

Example 3:

Sam creates an irrevocable trust that says that no distributions of trust property can be made back to him unless he is in a nursing home. He transfers $150,000 into the trust. Because there are still some circumstances under which the trust property can be distributed back to him, even though he's not in a nursing home now, this transfer is not considered a gift. A year later, he writes a $10,000 check from the trust to his grandson, as a college graduation gift. The gift to his grandson will be a disqualifying transfer subject to a 60-month lookback period. Should Sam apply for Medicaid within 60 months of that date, then assuming the state penalty divisor is $5,000, such gift will cause a two-month penalty period to run from the day he applies for Medicaid.

(NOTE: It may be possible for Sam to argue that the gift to his grandson was made exclusively for a purpose other than to qualify for Medicaid, which would eliminate the penalty. See page 140.)

What if you needed to receive income from the trust assets, to pay your living expenses, but still wanted to insulate the trust assets should you ever need to apply for Medicaid? In that case, what you should consider is an income-only trust. Let's take a look at how that works, now.

Income-Only Trusts

If you create an irrevocable trust and retain no rights to receive any distributions from this trust, you are deemed to have made a gift of the entire amount of assets you transferred into the trust. Since you have no access to the trust property, no part of the trust property is countable as an available asset of yours.

But what if your trust document permits the trustee to distribute trust *income* to you? So long as you can only receive the *income*—and the trustee can never distribute any portion of the trust *principal* to you—then the income is countable as your income, under the income rules discussed above, but the principal of the trust is still not countable as your property. So if you set up such a trust and transfer some part or all of your assets into the trust, once the five-year lookback period has passed the trust property will be ignored when the Medicaid eligibility department assesses your application.

Example:

Your attorney sets up an irrevocable income-only trust for you. You transfer $50,000 in cash into the trust. You have no right ever to get a distribution of any part of that $50,000, but the trustee does have the authority to distribute the income earned on that $50,000 back to you every quarter.

The full amount transferred into the trust—$50,000—is treated as a gift, just as if you gave it to a child of yours. As such, there is a penalty based on dividing the amount of the gift by your state "penalty divisor" figure. Assume the divisor is $5,000. Thus, $50,000 divided by $5,000 is 10, so that means there is a penalty period of 10 months. If you apply for Medicaid within five years of your transfer to the trust, this penalty period will have to be dealt with. Once the five-year period has passed, however, the gift will be ignored when you apply for Medicaid, and the assets inside the trust, no matter what their value is at that time, will also be ignored.

Dealing with Trust Income

Once you are in a nursing home, if you retained the right to all trust income, your trustee can change investments so as to minimize the distributions of income to you. Depending on the terms of the trust, it may also be possible for the trustee simply to stop distributing income to you. After all, every distribution of income to you must go directly to the nursing home, and once you are on Medicaid such distributions will serve only to reduce the amount that Medicaid would otherwise pay to the nursing home on your behalf. Your care will not change if the nursing home gets its fee entirely from the state under the Medicaid program, or if it gets part of its fee from your income and the balance from the Medicaid program. That's why it makes sense for your trustee to minimize or stop income distributions to you once you are in the nursing home.

Trigger Trust Option

As a way to deal with the "wasted income" problem discussed above, some trust documents state that if you are in a nursing home and receiving Medicaid, no income may be distributed to you. This is called a "trigger trust." Under former law, this was permitted but seems to have little utility, now. During the period you are entitled to receive the income, even if it is discretionary with the trustee, it is counted, even if you cannot demand a distribution. And if at some future time after the trust is established, your right to receive the income is terminated, you will be deemed to have made a gift on the termination date (of the present value of your income interest), causing a penalty period. In addition, some states have banned this option as being "against public policy."

Irrevocable Trusts vs. Outright Gifts

What if you have $100,000 of excess assets and must reduce your assets before you can qualify for Medicaid? What if you don't need nursing home care now, but may in, say, five years or more? Should you just give your children the money? Or transfer it into an irrevocable trust?

Here are some advantages of setting up and funding an irrevocable trust, as described above, vs. making the outright gift:

- the trust protects your assets while you are living, both from your children's creditors as well as your own;
- the trust permits you to serve as trustee, with one or more children named as successor trustees, so that you can continue to manage

and invest the assets as you see fit, so long as you are able to do so;

- the trust assets will not count against you when and if you ever need to apply for Medicaid, should you ever need nursing home care;
- the state cannot go after the trust assets after you die, under their "estate recovery" program, whereby they seek to be repaid for every dollar they spent on you while you were in the nursing home;
- the trust protects the assets from attack by a child's spouse, should they ever get divorced;
- the trust continues to allow you to control the ultimate disposition of the assets following your death, by retaining what is called a "testamentary limited power of appointment";
- the trust does not increase the Medicaid "lookback period" as compared to an outright gift (this used to be one reason people preferred outright gifts prior to the law being changed in February 2006);
- the trust can permit income to be distributed to you for life;
- it can permit "back door" distributions to family members should that be necessary down the road; and
- it permits a step-up in basis of gifted assets, saving income taxes for your children.

As you can see, there are many benefits to the trust compared to an outright gift to children. What are the drawbacks?

- A trust costs money to prepare (legal fees can be anywhere from $1,000 to $2,500 or more);
- it takes time to understand how it works;
- a new, separate bank account will have to be opened up in the name of the trust;
- a federal tax i.d. number must be obtained for the trust (although this is now easily done online);
- additional paperwork is involved for trust accounting; and
- a separate income tax return must be filed each year (Federal Form 1041).

Self-Settled Trusts

If you are under age 65 and considered disabled, a trust can be established for your benefit with your own assets that will not be counted for Medicaid eligibility purposes. The trust must be established by a parent, grandparent, legal guardian or a court, on your behalf. In order to qualify, the trust must contain a "payback" provision that requires the state to be reimbursed for all the Medicaid payments it made on your behalf during your lifetime.

Because the rules for such a trust are found in the federal statutes at 42 U.S.C. section 1396p(d)(4)(A), it is also known as a "(d)(4)(A)" trust.

Why would you do this? First of all, such a trust can *supplement* what the Medicaid program pays for, improving your lifestyle. For a list of typical items such a "supplemental needs" trust can pay for, see the list at the end of this chapter (p. 71).

Second, by qualifying for Medicaid coverage, your expenses will be paid for at the reduced "Medicaid rate," so even if your assets are ultimately used to reimburse the state, it will leave more of your assets to pass on to your family members (assuming the trust assets are not totally depleted by the reimbursement).

Pooled Trusts

A "pooled trust" is a trust fund set up by a non-profit organization within your state that holds funds of disabled individuals to be used to supplement their living expenses. The contributions of each disabled person are accounted for separately, but the assets of all contributors are invested and managed as a single "pooled" fund, hence the name.

Although it is an irrevocable trust, federal law has carved out an exception for pooled trusts from the normal trust rules discussed above. Accordingly, the transfer of assets *into* the trust is not considered a penalty-causing gift, and the assets *within* the trust are not counted as owned by the disabled person when that person applies for Medicaid. If the potential

Medicaid applicant is over age 65, however, some states will treat the transfer into the pooled trust as a disqualifying transfer. Thus, be sure to check your state rules before considering this option!

Because the rules for such a trust are found in the federal statutes at 42 U.S.C. section 1396p(d)(4)(C), it is also known as a "(d)(4)(C)" trust.

The important point is that the contribution of the disabled individual, while excluded for Medicaid purposes, can be used to pay for items that Medicaid does not pay for. For a list of typical items such a "supplemental needs" trust can pay for, see the list at the end of this chapter (p. 71).

Upon the Contributor's Death

It is important to note that upon the death of the disabled individual who contributed funds to the pooled trust, any remaining funds in that person's separate account must either be retained in the pooled trust for the benefit of others or used to pay back the state for any Medicaid outlays it made on behalf of the disabled individual during his or her lifetime. The balance of the account, if any, may then be paid to a named beneficiary (such as a family member) or left in the pooled trust to benefit others. Whether the full amount remaining at the contributor's death must be retained in the pooled trust, or only a certain percentage, depends on your state regulations. You can easily find this out by contacting the administrators of the pooled trust program in your state; you can find their contact information by doing an internet search under "pooled trust Florida" or whatever state you're in.

Reasons for Using Pooled Trusts

You might be thinking, if upon your family member's death all the remaining money in your family member's pooled trust account must either go to the state or remain inside the pooled trust, why do it? The reason is that without transferring the excess assets into a pooled trust, your disabled family member may have to spend all of his or her money on nursing home care until it's gone, and therefore have no money for supplemental care (see *Supplemental Needs: List*, page 71). With the pooled trust, the individual would qualify for Medicaid immediately, and yet the assets are still available to be spent for his or her supplemental care.

In addition, because a non-profit organization is managing the pooled trust and making appropriate distributions to each beneficiary, there is no need to find an individual or corporate trustee for the disabled individual's funds. Indeed, if the money involved is fairly modest, e.g., $50,000, it would be disproportionately costly to hire a trustee, but the money would still cause the disabled person to be disqualified from government benefits unless something is done with it. Finally, there is satisfaction in knowing that any amount of the trust account that remains at the death of your disabled family member will contribute to the pooled trust's support of other disabled and elderly individuals. Hence, the pooled trust could be the perfect solution; it is certainly a viable option to be considered when doing your Medicaid planning.

Trusts Created by Someone Else

A trust created by someone other than you or your spouse is known as a "third-party-created trust" or simply a "third-party trust." Different rules apply to these kinds of trusts than to a "self-created" trust that you set up for your own benefit. Here are the rules for third-party-created trusts.

If the trustee of a third-party-created trust has an obligation to pay for your "support" or "medical care" or similar terms, then the trust assets will be countable as your assets when you apply for Medicaid. The theory is that the trustee has a legal obligation to pay for your nursing home bills out of the trust property before Medicaid will pay for you. In such a case, all of the trust assets will have to be "spent down" to the level required before you will be eligible for Medicaid coverage.

"Supplemental Needs" Limitations

However, if the trustee is limited in paying for your care such that the trust property can only be used to "supplement" but not "supplant" benefits otherwise available to you, then such a trust generally will not be a countable asset for Medicaid eligibility purposes. The theory is that if the trustee is barred from making distributions that would reduce or replace what Medicaid already pays for, the trust assets are not considered to be "available" to you— and therefore are non-countable—for Medicaid eligibility purposes.

In many states, if the trustee is given broad "sole and absolute discretion" whether or not to distribute anything to you, then the trust assets are not countable for Medicaid purposes. The theory is that since you have no legal right to force the trustee to distribute anything to you, the assets cannot be counted as available to you.

Because these types of trusts state that they are only to "supplement" benefits otherwise available to—or pay for the "special needs" of—a disabled beneficiary, they have become known among attorneys as "supplemental needs trusts" or "special needs trusts."

You'll definitely need the assistance of a skilled elder law attorney if you find that you wish to set up a trust for the benefit of someone other than yourself who is planning on applying for—or who is already receiving—Medicaid or other governmental assistance.

Trusts Created Within a Spouse's Will

Under federal law, if Spouse A creates a trust for the benefit of Spouse B, the trust is nonetheless treated as if created by Spouse B for his or her own benefit. As such, the trust is treated as a self-settled trust, described above, with the result that in most cases all of the trust assets will be considered to be available to Spouse B.

One exception to the above rule is that if a trust is created *within the will* of a deceased spouse for the benefit of the surviving spouse, the trust assets are *not* countable as assets of the surviving spouse, assuming certain requirements are met. Basically, such a trust will be treated as a "third-party-created" trust, described above, and should therefore include supplemental needs language.

Example:

Marsha goes to her attorney to draw up a will for her that leaves all of her assets in a trust for the benefit of her husband, Louis, who is residing in a nursing home. The trust states that distributions can only be made—in the discretion of the trustee—for the supplemental needs of Louis, and no distributions can be made that would reduce any government benefits he would otherwise be entitled to receive. Upon Marsha's death, her assets flow into this trust and are held for the benefit of Louis without causing him to be disqualified from Medicaid. (See, however, *Elective Share Problem*, page 150.)

This type of trust is called by lawyers a "testamentary" trust because it is created within a Last Will and Testament, an old-fashioned expression for a will.

Supplemental Needs: List

"Supplemental needs" are those needs of a nursing home resident or other disabled individual that are not covered by Medicaid or Medicare, yet are important in making life better for the individual. Here is only a partial list of such items:

- supplemental nursing or geriatric care
- alternative medical therapies
- physician specialists if not covered by Medicaid
- dental work not covered by Medicaid, including anesthesia
- massage sessions
- haircuts and salon services
- over-the-counter medications (including vitamins and herbs, etc.)
- non-food grocery items
- personal assistance not covered by Medicaid
- taxi cab rides and other travel expenses to visit family members
- a specially equipped auto or van
- furniture, home furnishings
- clothing
- cell phone and service costs
- vacation trips (including a personal assistant to facilitate the trip)
- entertainment (large TV for the room, etc.)
- upgrade cost for a private room (Medicaid only pays for a semi-private room)
- attorney fees

Chapter 10

STRATEGIES TO QUALIFY

Hiding Assets: Don't Do It!

Good Medicaid planning does not rely on hiding assets or any other illegal means. When you fill out the application to receive Medicaid benefits, "forgetting" to disclose certain assets you own or not disclosing gifts you have made to family members is not a good idea. This is called **Medicaid fraud** and anyone convicted of this:

- is liable to the federal government for damages ranging from two to three times the amount of benefits received wrongfully,
- is liable for penalties of $5,000 to $10,000 for each false claim submitted,
- is liable to the federal government for the costs of bringing the action against such person,
- is subject to a *criminal* penalty of up to one year in prison and a $10,000 fine, and
- may be barred from receiving Medicaid for up to one year.

Further, the state you live in will have its *own* statute related to your illegal act, with its own penalties in addition to those above.

Finally, anyone who files suit against you on behalf of the government for Medicaid fraud is rewarded with a 15-30% "cut" of the penalties ultimately imposed on you, so you better be on good terms with your neighbors and relatives!

As you can see, hiding assets is not to be recommended! With good planning, you will be able to qualify for Medicaid without committing fraud against the government.

Spenddown

"Spend down" is what you do when you have too many resources, i.e., too much money, and you are told that you must "spend down" your assets before you will be eligible for Medicaid coverage. Those excess assets are called your "spenddown" amount.

The classic "spend down" technique is to pay for your nursing home bill out of your own assets until you have reduced your life savings to the point that you qualify for Medicaid coverage of those bills.

In most cases, however, you do not have to spend anything. Instead you can essentially convert an asset that is countable into one that is not countable. The idea is that instead of spending your money on something that Medicaid can ultimately pay for, you pay for something that will benefit you or your family yet not be considered a gift or a countable asset.

There are some very smart ways to spend down. The next section of this book describes these techniques in detail.

Converting Countable Assets to Non-Countable

Home Improvements

Since your home is an excluded asset, any improvements you make to your home are also excluded. Assuming you are able to pass your house on to your children following your death, then the money you put into improvements will be money saved. Have you delayed repairing your roof? Finishing your basement? Replacing your out-of-date kitchen? Updating your heating/air-conditioning system? Paving your driveway? All of these cost thousands of dollars. By investing in your home in these ways, you are sheltering your money while reducing your "Medicaid-countable" assets at the same time.

Adding an addition on to your house is another possibility, especially if this permits a child of yours to move into your house (see *Caretaker Child,* page 139).

New Home, Bigger Home

An alternative to improving your home is to sell your older, smaller home and move into a newer and/or larger home. Remember that your equity in the home cannot exceed $500,000 (which can be increased to as much as $750,000 under federal law, *if* the state you are in so chooses). Under Internal Revenue Code section 121 you are able to sell your home and shelter up to $250,000 of the capital gains ($500,000 if you are married at the time of the sale). The old rules of being over age 55, and it being a once-in-a-lifetime benefit, no longer apply. Now, you can qualify for this tax sheltering device every two years. The only rule is that you must have resided in the house as your primary residence for at least two of the previous five years.

Example 1:

Sarah has $250,000 in bank accounts and CDs and lives in a house valued at $250,000. She does not need nursing home care at this point, but is concerned about the future. Her daughter, Molly, lives nearby and has expressed her willingness to move in with her mother to care for her. Sarah decides to sell her house and purchase one for $500,000, large enough for Sarah and Molly to live comfortably. After two years, Sarah deeds the house to her daughter, as a gift. Because of the *Caretaker Child* exception (page 139), there are no Medicaid gift penalties that apply (but there could be *state gift tax* if you live in one of the gift tax states, discussed on page 56). Should Sarah need nursing home care in the future, she will no longer have to worry about losing her house following her death, since she has already gotten it out of her name and into her daughter's name, and reduced her countable assets at the same time. Accordingly, Sarah should immediately be able to qualify for Medicaid.

Example 2:

Gus has $150,000 in countable assets and lives in an apartment. Gus's son, Dave, is married and lives in another state. Gus decides to invest his $150,000 in an addition to be built onto Dave's house. Gus then moves into the addition. Gus doesn't worry about whether Dave will "take care of" Gus for at least two years (see the *Caretaker Child* exception (page 139)), because they created the deed of Gus's interest in the house so that it is jointly owned, with a "right of survivorship" to his son, Dave, and Dave's wife. This guarantees that upon Gus's death, his interest in the house will automatically pass to his son and daughter-in-law. By writing the deed this way, Gus's interest passes outside of his probate estate, which means that most states will not be able to make a claim for "estate recovery" against the son's house following Gus's death. (See further discussion of *Estate Recovery*, page 155.)

If you are single, you must still be living in the community for some period of time for this to work. If you are already in the nursing home, it is too late to purchase a larger or more expensive home. The basis for excluding the home is your intent to "return" to your old residence. If you never lived in a house, how can you argue you have the intent to "return" to that house? If you are married, however, it is perfectly allowable for your spouse in the community to purchase and move into a larger or more expensive house.

Example:

Henry and Maude have $200,000 in countable assets and a home worth $150,000. Maude has to move into a nursing home, so Henry sells the old home and purchases a smaller but more expensive home for $250,000. That leaves the couple $100,000, which is sheltered by the CSRA of $101,640 allowed to Henry. Maude is now eligible for Medicaid coverage and should apply immediately.

Personal Property

Since all personal property is excluded, it makes sense to "upgrade" one's clothes, shoes, sheets, towels, TV set (buy that big-screen TV you've had your eye on), audio components, computer system, musical instruments (buy a $10,000 piano), etc. However, be careful not to get carried away. As discussed above on page 38, spending too much on art objects or jewelry may lead the Medicaid eligibility workers to decide that such purchases are not excluded but are countable investment assets. If so, you haven't lost anything, but you haven't gained anything either: You've taken countable cash and simply moved it into a different form of countable asset, still leaving you with too many assets.

New Auto, Bigger Auto

Under the new regulations discussed above (p. 38), one automobile— of any value—will be excluded if it is used for your transportation or that of a member of your household. In other words, even if you cannot drive, the auto will be excluded if it is owned by you and used to drive you or a member of your household around. Note that if a family member or hired driver resides outside of your home but uses the auto to provide you *or another household member* with transportation, it will still be excluded.

Thus, purchasing a new car or larger car (e.g., one that will accommodate a wheelchair or electric mobility scooter) is a good way to move assets from the countable column to the non-countable column. Oftentimes the older generation has held onto an older vehicle, since they have developed admirable traits of frugality. However, now is the time to sell or trade-in the old model for a new one, since it will enable them to shelter a significant amount of cash. It may make sense to purchase a van that is wheelchair accessible.

Once again, be wary of going out and purchasing a Ferrari or Rolls-Royce: The Medicaid workers may consider that to be an investment, and instead of sheltering the $25,000-$30,000 you might have sheltered had you purchased a more ordinary Toyota or Honda, you wind up sheltering none of your cash! Attorneys have an expression that applies in these cases: "Pigs get fat, but hogs get slaughtered!" So, yes, go ahead and be shrewd, take advantage of every available legal opportunity, but just don't get greedy!

Funeral/Burial Expenses

Pre-pay these expenses (see *Funeral and Burial Funds,* page 39). If you spend down all your assets to qualify for Medicaid, then your family will have to pay for your funeral and burial out of their own pockets. So it makes more sense for you to pre-pay these expenses yourself, out of your own assets. It will reduce your otherwise countable assets and spare your family from having to pay this large expense following your death.

With the average cost of a funeral and burial now hovering around $8,500, this is a good way to spend down your excess funds. If you are married, since you can pay not only for yourself but also for your spouse, this alone can usually protect at least $17,000. If you are willing to prepay for the burial spaces of other family members, you should go ahead and do that also (see p. 40, above). Once again, this can permit you to pay for something that will benefit your family yet not be considered a gift or a countable asset. Depending on how many of your family members you are willing to prepay this for—and the size of your family—this can easily allow you to protect an additional $10,000 - $20,000 in otherwise countable assets.

Income-Producing Property

If the unlimited exclusion for income-producing property is available in your state (see discussion on page 85), this could be one of the best possible strategies to convert countable assets to non-countable. Simply invest the excess cash into rental real estate.

For example, an unmarried individual could have $2,000 in the bank, own his own home, and also own a house worth $350,000 that is rented out, and still qualify for Medicaid. Note that the net income generated by the rental property would be countable, so you can reach a point where although the rental property is excluded, it generates so much income that your total income exceeds the full cost of the nursing home. So as a practical matter, even though the property is not counted, Medicaid won't be available to you, because your income will equal or exceed the nursing home bill, leaving nothing for Medicaid to pay!

Annuities

Certain types of annuities are non-countable for Medicaid eligibility purposes. Because of the importance and complexity of the use of annuities in Medicaid planning, please see the separate detailed discussion of *Annuities* on page 105.

Converting Non-Countable Assets to Countable

There is one situation where you may want to *increase* the amount of your countable assets: if you are a married couple where one spouse is about to enter a nursing home and your state calculates the CSRA using the 50% method (see *Fifty Percent States*, page 43). In such case, in order to maximize the CSRA protection, your goal should be to have total countable assets (owned by husband, wife, or joint) at least equal to twice the CSRA. Currently, the CSRA is $101,640, so your goal should be to have approximately $200,000 in countable assets at the time of the "snapshot" (i.e., the date the first spouse enters the nursing home). (See discussion of the *"Snapshot" Rule*, page 42.)

What if you have only $100,000 in countable assets? Unless you do something, the Community Spouse will only be able to protect half of that—$50,000—and the nursing home spouse will have to spend down the balance to $2,000, i.e., spend $48,000.

But if you own a house, there is a way to increase the CSRA. The house is normally an excluded asset and won't count toward your $200,000 goal. However, if the house is inside a revocable ("living") trust, then it *is* a countable asset as to the person with the power to revoke the trust. So if you already have a revocable trust, contact your attorney to deed the house into the name of the trust, or have your attorney create a revocable trust specifically for this purpose and then deed the house into the name of the trust. This must be done before either spouse has moved into a nursing home, because the countable assets must be increased *before* the "snapshot" date.

Example:

John and Alice have $100,000 of countable assets and a house worth $200,000. If Alice enters the nursing home now, John will be able to keep and protect 50% of their countable assets, i.e., $50,000, as the CSRA. Alice can only keep $2,000, so the couple must figure out how to spend down or otherwise deplete the balance of $48,000.

Instead, John and Alice have their lawyer create a revocable trust and deed the house into the trust prior to Alice entering the nursing home. Since the home is now titled in the name of the trust, it is a countable asset, so their countable assets have just increased to $300,000.

As soon as Alice enters the nursing home, they apply for Medicaid. A "snapshot" of their assets is taken for purposes of calculating the CSRA. The CSRA calculation goes like this: Community Spouse can protect 50% of the couple's countable assets, up to the maximum of $101,640. Fifty percent of $300,000 is $150,000, so John can retain the full $101,640 as the CSRA. Of course, since he only has $100,000 of countable assets other than the house, that's what he will really be protecting.

After the Medicaid application and determination of the CSRA, here's what John and Alice have:

Countable assets	$300,000
CSRA exclusion (John)	(101,640)
Nursing home spouse exclusion (Alice)	(2,000)
Spenddown amount	$196,360

But rather than spending down the $196,360, the trustee of the revocable trust (which should be the Community Spouse) simply deeds the house out of the trust back into the name of the Community Spouse (it's a good idea, for estate recovery purposes, to keep the nursing home spouse's name off the house). Once the house is titled again in John's name, it immediately converts back into an excluded asset, leaving him with protected assets of $100,000. Since the snapshot is only done once, the Community Spouse does not have to refigure the CSRA and therefore he can keep his full $100,000 even after this transfer out of the trust.

After the house is deeded out of the trust, here's what John and Alice have:

Excluded value of their home	-0-
Countable assets	$100,000
CSRA exclusion (John)	(101,640)
	-0-

As you can see, this leaves Alice with $-0-, so when she applies for Medicaid, she will immediately qualify. **Result:** John gets to keep not just $50,000, but $100,000, fully doubling his protected assets!

NOTE: This technique is not required in any of the so-called "100% states" (discussed above). These states permit the Community Spouse to protect the full "maximum" CSRA even if the countable assets are less than twice that amount. So there would be no point in trying to increase the countable assets just prior to the "snapshot" date for any couple living in one of these states. Furthermore, it will only make sense to do if the total of the combined countable assets of a couple is *greater* than the minimum CSRA ($20,328) and *less than* two times the maximum amount (2 x $101,640= $203,280). So if a couple's countable assets exceed $203,280, then in all states, the Community Spouse will be able to protect the full $101,640.

Decreasing the Home Equity Amount

If your home is above the state limit (assume the state has not enacted an increased limit above $500,000), in order for the home to be excluded you will need to reduce your equity interest. How can you do that?

Here are some ways, both good and bad:

- **Take out a reverse mortgage:** Taking out a reverse mortgage on the house is not a good idea: If there is a Community Spouse living in the home, the home is excluded no matter what it is worth, so this is not needed. If there is no Community Spouse, a reverse mortgage cannot be obtained if the owner does not live in the house. If the owner takes out a reverse mortgage and then has to move to a nursing home, the mortgage must be paid off within one year of the owner moving out. That will often force a sale of the house, thereby exposing the entire amount of equity to nursing home costs.

- **Obtain a home equity loan:** How will the owner in the nursing home pay back the loan? Once on Medicaid, the owner will not be permitted to divert income to pay the loan. Thus, this is impractical unless other family members are willing to carry the loan or pay it off, possibly in exchange for an ownership interest in the house. If the equity is just a little over $500,000, then maybe this can be a reasonable option to explore, to make sure the house is excluded so the owner can receive (or continued to receive) Medicaid coverage.

- **Deed a small percentage of the house to a family member:** Another option is to transfer a small percentage ownership interest in the house to one or more children. Although this will be a gift, the penalty period may be well worth it, if it permits you to qualify for

Medicaid. In addition, if you are able to wait five years before applying for Medicaid, then the gift cannot count against you.

NOTE: Some states ignore the actual wording of the deed and deem a transfer of any percentage to one other person as if you transferred 50%! Thus, you would be deemed to have a made a very large gift, incurring a lengthy penalty. As you can see, deeding an interest in your home (to a child, for example) is not something to be done casually or without complete understanding of the Medicaid rules as well as the other legal consequences of adding someone to your deed.

- **Lend Money to a Family Member:** The homeowner could borrow money from a family member in exchange for giving them a security interest in the house, thereby reducing the equity below the $500,000 value. The borrowed money can then be spent down or gifted back to family members. Be sure to have the debt recorded at the local county real estate recorder's office.

Transferring Excluded Assets

As discussed above, certain assets you own are not countable for purposes of determining if you can qualify for Medicaid. These items include the furniture and furnishings in your home, your auto, personal jewelry, etc. Because these items are "excluded," you can transfer any of them without incurring a penalty period. These excluded assets are simply not considered "assets" for purposes of the transfer penalty rules.

Be careful of running out and buying, say, a $150,000 Rolls-Royce, or expensive artwork, antiques or jewelry, and then immediately transferring title to your children. Such items are *not* excluded, because (i) the Rolls was not used for your transportation, and (ii) the artwork, antiques and jewelry were not either personal property found in or near your home, that are used on a regular basis, or items needed by you for maintenance, use and occupancy of your premises as a home. In short, such personal items will be deemed investments and therefore countable.

IRAs

The IRA, 401(k), 403(b), etc., ("retirement plan") assets of the Medicaid applicant (single or married) are counted the same as cash. The plan assets of the Community Spouse may or may not be countable, depending on your state law. However, if the plan assets are countable, it is usually possible to convert the plan assets into a fixed, irrevocable stream of annuity payments, starting immediately, typically by transferring the non-IRA retirement plan assets into an Individual Retirement Annuity under Internal Revenue Code section 408 or 408A. By converting the plan to that of a fixed immediate annuity, the annuity rules discussed below apply (see *Annuities*, page 105), making the plan assets immediately non-countable. *In addition, the state payback rules do not apply!* (The federal statute carved out an exception to the requirement of naming the state as beneficiary for annuities purchased with proceeds of IRAs (see *Payback to State*, page 109).)

Of course, you still have to satisfy the minimum distribution requirements of the Internal Revenue Code, so be sure to set the annuity payments so that the person receiving the payments is certain to receive at least the minimum amount under these rules (found under Internal Revenue Code section 401(a)(9)). If the annuity payments are less than the minimum required amount under these income tax rules, there is a hefty 50% tax on the amount you were supposed to withdraw but didn't, i.e., the shortfall.

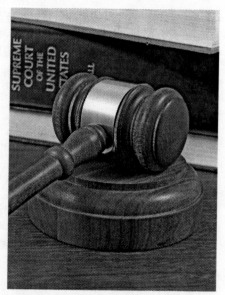

Because IRAs and similar retirement plan assets (known as "qualified plan" assets) will be subject to income taxation once the assets are withdrawn or paid to a beneficiary, you should try to take out the money from such a plan over more than one calendar year, if possible, so as to spread the income over two tax years. In most cases, this will save taxes.

Income-Producing Property

Many states completely exclude any property that generates income on a monthly basis. They will count the income, of course, but not the underlying property that generates the income. The term "property" as used in this context means not only real estate but other "tangible" personal property (i.e., something you can put your hands on, like jewelry, furniture, or autos, as opposed to bank account interest, dividends from stocks, bonds, etc.). So although a bank CD generates income, the CD is not considered "property," so this rule will not exclude the CD.

/// **Example:**

Maude has $400,000 in the bank, invested in stocks, bonds, and her savings and checking accounts. Because Maude is single, she is only permitted to retain $2,000 of cash. Her son, using his power of attorney, uses all of Maude's assets to purchase two $200,000 condos, and then rents them out to tenants. He is allowed to pay himself a management fee (or, if he does not want to do this job, he can hire a management company to handle all of the management and administrative work involved in keeping the units rented, calling the plumber on the weekend, etc.). All management fees, assessments, real estate taxes, and utility costs not payable by the tenants may be subtracted from the gross rent. The net rent must be paid to the nursing home. As long as the total net rental income is less than the cost of the nursing home, Medicaid will pick up the difference. The deed is structured so that upon Maude's death it is out of her estate, so as to avoid estate recovery. In states that limit estate recovery to the "probate" estate, the property should be titled in such manner as to pass automatically to a new owner upon the Medicaid applicant's death. So Maude should consider titling the house jointly with her son with "rights of survivorship," so that upon Maude's death it passes automatically to the son, avoiding probate and avoiding the state's ability to recover its Medicaid expenditures. Similar results may be obtained using a Ladybird Deed (see page 100)), if it is available *///* in Maude's state.

"Just Say No" (Spousal Refusal to Support)

Under the federal Medicaid statutes, if the Community Spouse simply refuses to pay for the nursing home care of the ill spouse, the state cannot consider the assets of the Community Spouse in determining the Medicaid eligibility of the nursing home spouse, if:

(i) the nursing home spouse has assigned to the state any rights to support from the Community Spouse; or

(ii) the nursing home spouse is unable to execute such an assignment due to a physical or mental disability; or

(iii) the state determines that denial of eligibility would work an "undue hardship."

Example:

Mrs. Smith, who now lives in a nursing home in New York, signs a short document assigning her spousal support rights to the State of New York. At the same time, Mr. Smith signs another short document stating that he refuses to contribute to the support of his wife anymore. As a result, *only the assets of Mrs. Smith* may be counted in determining whether she is eligible for Medicaid. Mr. Smith may have $1 million in the bank, but once these two documents are signed, those assets cannot be considered for Medicaid eligibility purposes.

While certain states (such as New York) have routinely allowed this procedure, others have not. A recent federal court decision (*Morenz v. Wilson-Coker*, 415 F. 3d 230 (2nd Cir. 2005)) held that Connecticut, which claimed that it did not allow "spousal refusal," *must* follow the federal law and permit this procedure.

Accordingly, even if your state has not allowed the "Just Say No" procedure in the past, you may want to consider having your attorney bring a lawsuit to enforce it in your state. A lot of money could be at stake, and the cost of the legal work may be money well spent. Based on the clear language of this case, you have an extremely good chance of winning!

Personal Services Contract

It may come as a shock to most people to find out that adult children are not legally obligated to care for their elderly parents. While there may be a *moral* obligation for a child to care for those folks who changed his diapers and paid for his college education, there is no legal obligation to do so.

Thus, it may be a good way to reduce a parent's countable assets by having the children charge the parent for any caregiving the child performs for the parent.

A child or other family member is permitted to contract with the parent to provide personal care to the parent. Such payments will help to deplete the parent's countable assets without causing imposition of a penalty. After all, as long as the payments are reasonable and in line with the going rate for similar services provided by commercial companies in the same general geographic area, the parent is getting fair value for his or her money.

Since all such contracts will be scrutinized by the Medicaid agency in your state, be sure to follow the following guidelines:

- Prepare a written contract prior to the delivery of the personal care services
- Detail what types of services are included and what are excluded (e.g., non-medical care only; cooking meals; light housekeeping; assistance with activities of daily living)
- Have the parent and the person agreeing to perform the services both sign the contract (if the parent is unable to sign due to mental incapacity, have the agent under a durable power of attorney sign on the parent's behalf)
- Have all signatures notarized at the time of signing
- Date the contract
- Make sure that the rate charged is comparable to locally available equivalent commercial rates. Call two or three local elder care companies to get a good idea of what is fair and reasonable for the type of services to be provided under the contract. If the rate charged exceeds the going rate by a significant amount, the Medicaid workers

may decide that it's really a hidden gift, and impose a penalty. After all, if your parent can hire a commercial caregiver at $20/hour, and you're charging $50/hour, then the $30/hour rate difference is really a gift to you from your parent.

- Keep an accurate log of all services performed and money received, after the contract is signed.

Life Care Contract

Some states permit a parent to pay a child a lump sum in advance, for life care. Such a "Life Care Contract" is more difficult to prepare and calculate, since the amount and duration of care will depend on the age, health, and needs of the parent, going forward for many years. However, the advantage of such a contract is that it permits the immediate depletion of the parent's countable assets without it being a penalty-causing gift. As such, if this is permitted in your state, it is something you may want to discuss with your elder law attorney.

Unfortunately, some states do not recognize such a contract, deeming any money transferred under such a contract to be countable resources or a penalty-causing gift.

Income Taxes/Reporting Requirements

Any time one person hires another person to do something, and pays them, Uncle Sam is going to want a piece of the money changing hands. Accordingly, if you are going to be paid for caring for a parent, be sure you have checked with your accountant regarding the following issues:

- Your status as either an "employee" or an "independent contractor" (Most domestic workers and cleaning people are considered employees, particularly if they only have one employer.)
- Income tax withholding (state and federal)
- Social Security withholding
- Medicare withholding
- FUTA (Federal Unemployment Tax Act) requirements
- IRS Forms W-2 and W-4

Liquidating Assets

In many of the planning techniques discussed in this book you must either gift assets to another family member or sell the asset and convert it to another type of asset. There may be specific consequences to such gifts or sales you should be aware of, so that you can decide which assets should be liquidated first.

For example, if you need to cash out an annuity, there may be penalties if this is done within the first few years of purchase. You need to take a look at the original contract terms. Alternatively, ask the broker or agent who sold you the annuity to find this out.

Real Estate

For Medicaid planning purposes, there are really two categories of real estate, each requiring different treatment. The first applies only to your home—your personal residence. As discussed above, your home is an excluded resource if your equity interest is below $500,000 (page 35). Accordingly, the only reason to transfer your interest in your home, if you are applying for Medicaid, is so that upon your death, you will not own it, thereby protecting it from estate recovery.

Any other real estate you own will be a countable asset, and in order to qualify for Medicaid if you are unmarried, you will have to sell it and deal with the proceeds, or gift it away. If you are married, the non-home real estate can certainly form part of the CSRA (depending on its value), but that will leave little cash for the Community Spouse, so it usually will have to be sold.

If you decide not to transfer your entire interest in a parcel of real estate, but instead to add the name of an additional owner to your deed (e.g., a child of yours), you need to be aware that some states ignore the real estate ownership rules and apply a different rule for Medicaid eligibility purposes when a person is added to a deed. See discussion on page 95 (*Add Child's Name to Deed*).

Another difference between residential and non-residential property is that there is a capital gains tax exclusion that only applies to a sale of the personal residence. Essentially, you can exclude up to $250,000 ($500,000 if married and filing jointly) of capital gains from a sale of your home, if you lived there at least two of the previous five years. If the property you're selling is not your home, you will face a capital gains tax of 15% on the difference between what you receive when you sell the property, and what you paid for it (increased by any capital improvements). Be sure to check with your accountant, so you will be prepared for any resulting tax!

CDs

If a bank or broker-issued certificate of deposit ("CD") is one of the assets that is causing you to be disqualified from the Medicaid program, you will have no choice but to either transfer it or cash it in. Although there is typically a penalty if you cash in a CD prior to its maturity date, that cost will be negligible compared to the cost of the nursing home if it causes you to lose Medicaid coverage for another month!

Frequently, however, you do not need to cash in the CD. You can simply transfer the ownership to another family member. Since this is not a "withdrawal" of the funds from the bank or brokerage, there is no penalty imposed. When considering what assets should be transferred as part of a gifting program, consider what CDs you can keep and what should be transferred, and finally what must be cashed out. Be sure to consider the amount of any early withdrawal penalty when calculating your "spenddown."

Questionable Techniques

Single Premium No-Cash Irrevocable Life Insurance

A number of enterprising insurance companies have recently begun promoting single pay, no cash value, irrevocable, non-cancelable, non-assignable, non-amendable life insurance policies. These are issued with no or only minimal medical examinations.

While there are different variations in each company's product, the basic idea is the same: since only the cash value of life insurance is a countable asset, then so long as the policy states that there is *no* cash value, the entire value of the policy is non-countable for Medicaid purposes.

While the foregoing is true, these products fail for one simple reason: the purchase of such a life insurance policy is a gift, resulting in a penalty period. This is so because the insured/Medicaid applicant transfers money and receives nothing in return: the insured "owner" of the policy cannot gain access to the cash value since there is none, cannot change the beneficiary designations, and cannot transfer or cancel the policy. The only way that a transfer is not penalized as a gift is if there is something that the person making the transfer gets back in return for the cash paid to the company issuing the product. Since the policy beneficiaries are the only individuals who will benefit from the life insurance (i.e., they receive the proceeds or face value of the policy upon the insured's death), the purchase of the policy is an immediate gift to those family members. Although the insured may be listed as the "owner" of the policy, in reality the beneficiaries are the owners, since the insured retains no control over the terms of the policy once it is paid for.

So, the bottom line is, yes, the single premium no cash value, irrevocable life insurance policy is not a countable asset for Medicaid purposes, but purchasing such a policy will almost certainly be deemed a penalty-causing gift by the Medicaid agency in your state.

Family Limited Partnership

A "family limited partnership" ("FLP") is a legal partnership where only family members are the partners. For example, parent and children all invest in owning an apartment building, and a partnership agreement is drawn up indicating what percentage of the profits each partner will be entitled to receive, what rights each partner has in managing the partnership, etc.

Such a legal entity is widely used in business investments, and within the last 15 years or so has also become popular for estate planning purposes as a way of reducing the value of a partner's taxable estate, so as to reduce or eliminate estate taxes.

For Medicaid planning purposes, however, use of a family limited partnership is risky because many states have taken the position that such an investment is simply a way to make gifts to family members. As such, caution is urged before this technique is to be followed.

Retroactive Personal Services Contract

Once a child finds out about the ability to charge a parent for personal services, the child typically says, *"Gee, well I've been taking care of Mom for the last three years and never charged her a dime! Can't I get paid for that, now?"*

Unfortunately, the general rule is that it is too late to charge the parent for services rendered by the child at this point, once the services have been performed without a written contract in place. The Medicaid regulations assume that such caregiving was performed for "love and affection" unless there was a contract in place *in advance* of the performance of such services.

Self-Canceling Installment Notes ("SCIN")

If a parent lends money to a child, and the child signs a promissory note to repay the loan over time with monthly payments, only the stream of payments is counted—as income—when the parent applies for Medicaid. Assuming the loan cannot be canceled, assigned or sold to someone else, the parent has no rights in the money once it is loaned, so the money that was loaned is no longer a countable asset.

That sounds like a good result, but there is a problem with this arrangement: If the parent dies before the note is fully paid off, the balance due is part of the parent's probate estate and the state could now file a claim against that money for all the Medicaid payments it made on behalf of the parent. (This is discussed more fully at *Estate Recovery,* page 155.)

To avoid having the unpaid balance of the note included in the probate estate of the lender/parent—and therefore subject to estate recovery—attorneys came up the idea of simply having the note cancel upon the lender's death.

Unfortunately, over the last few years many states had banned the use of a self-canceling installment note, and the Deficit Reduction Act of 2005 put the final nail in the coffin by requiring all promissory notes to prohibit cancellation upon the death of the lender if the lender wants to avoid having the *loan* treated as it were a *gift.*

Chapter 11

THE HOME: PLANNING IDEAS

The Goal

For most people, the personal residence is the single largest investment they have. For people considering Medicaid to cover long-term care costs, it is almost always the biggest asset to deal with.

The home occupies a unique position in Medicaid planning not only because of its value, but because it is an excluded asset while the Medicaid recipient is living, but it becomes subject to estate recovery following the recipient's death. Thus, dealing with the home is usually not an issue related to *qualifying* for Medicaid, but rather one of protecting the home against estate recovery following the death of the nursing home resident/Medicaid recipient. (See *Estate Recovery*, page 155.)

> The goal, therefore, is to make sure that the Medicaid recipient has no interest in the home upon death or at least an interest that cannot be reached by the estate recovery program of your state. How best to do that, and the various consequences of each option, will be the topic of this chapter. (Also review Case Study #2 for an additional discussion of these ideas.)

Do Nothing

If the parent/Medicaid recipient still owns the house upon entering the nursing home, it is important to remember that the house will not have to be sold to pay nursing home expenses. Unfortunately, some people, afraid that the home will have to be sold, make transfers that are ill-advised or borrow against the house and pay privately for long-term care, when Medicaid could have paid for the care of the homeowner, saving the family thousands of dollars.

Outright Transfer to Children

An obvious option is to deed the home from the parent's name to the child's or children's names. This is a gift for both gift tax and Medicaid eligibility purposes.

Medicaid Gift

As discussed above, a gift to a child is ordinarily a disqualifying transfer for Medicaid eligibility purposes. Take the current state divisor figure for your state (published by your state) and divide it into the amount of the gift to calculate the number of months of the penalty period.

Example:

Bobby Lee deeds her Tennessee house to her son, when it is valued at $250,000. Under Tennessee rules, the state "divisor" is $3,394, so this transfer just caused Bobby Lee a penalty of 73.7 months! Since this is longer than the lookback period of 60 months, she will be better off not to apply for Medicaid until after the 60-month period has expired.

In addition to the gift tax and Medicaid penalty issues, deeding the house to one or more children means that you no longer own your own house. Your children can boot you out at any time! Now of course that's unlikely, but the fact remains that if a child is sued or divorced, "your" house—which is now really your *child's* house—can be subject to a forced sale to satisfy the creditor or divorcing spouse, leaving you out on the street. So while this technique may work in certain family situations, just be sure you know the risks and costs and go into it with your eyes open.

Add Child's Name to Deed

A gift of real estate is accomplished by signing a deed of the property into the name of the new owner. That seems self-evident, and anyone who has ever bought a house is familiar with how property is transferred. However, it is not generally understood that merely *adding* a person's name to your own, on a deed, is also a gift. Attorneys are always amazed at the number of times clients tell them something like, *"We added our son's name to the deed, so that we can avoid probate on our deaths."* If the attorney asks the client if he or she filed a gift tax return, the client will be incredulous: *"Gift tax return? For what?"*

So let me set the record straight: When you add a person's name to a deed you have made a gift to that person, equal to 50% of the fair market value of the property on the date the deed was signed. Why is that? Because once you sign the deed, the individual whose name you added to the deed is a joint owner of that property with you, and can immediately sell or give away their half of the property, or petition the court to "partition" (i.e., divide) the property, separating out their half.

There is a presumption that if no percentage ownership is set forth in the deed, all listed co-owners own the real estate equally. If you wish to make a gift of a smaller percentage interest in the property, then you must spell that out in the deed: *"I hereby transfer to John Smith of Yorkville, NY, a five percent (5%) undivided interest in the following property: (etc.)"* In this case, your ownership interest dropped from 100% to 95%, and you made a gift of 5% to John Smith.

Adding the name of one or more of your children to your deed can also prevent estate recovery against your house following your death *if* (i) your state does not have an "expanded definition" of estate recovery that includes joint property (see page 157) and (ii) the deed titles all owners as "joint tenants with right of survivorship" (sometimes abbreviated as "JTWROS").

The consequences of adding one or more children to a deed are the following:

Gift Value

In many states, adding one child to a deed is deemed a gift of 1/2 of the value of the house; adding two children is deemed a gift of 2/3 of the value of the house; etc. However, in some states that is merely a *presumption* that applies unless the deed language states otherwise. If that is the case in your state, you can deed a tiny percentage (e.g., 1%) to one or more children, and still attach the right of survivorship to accomplish your goals without incurring a large gift. (Your attorney may have to research this, as this is a new concept for many attorneys.) The advantages of reducing the size of the gift are threefold: (i) it reduces the penalty period should you need to apply for Medicaid within the lookback period after making the gift; (ii) it reduces the amount of gift tax in those states with their own gift tax; and (iii) it minimizes the percent of your house that would be subject to your child's creditors.

Exposure to Child's Creditors

Once a child is on the deed, the child's interest in your house is an asset of the child's, and therefore subject to attachment and forced sale should the child be sued or divorced. Unless you can make a transfer of a tiny percentage as discussed above, your ability to remain in the house may be jeopardized if you add one or more children to the deed.

Loss of Control

Once you add children to the deed, you cannot sell or refinance the house without the signature of all the owners, i.e., you would need to obtain the signatures of all the children. Worse, what if one of the children predeceased you? Then you'd need to figure out who the successor in interest to the deceased child is—it could be the deceased child's spouse or a bunch of minor grandchildren, etc.

Transfer to Children, Keep Life Estate

An alternative method of getting the house out of your name at death, but still keeping it in your name during life so you continue to control it and can't be forced out by a creditor of your child, is to keep a life estate in the house. What this means is that you transfer the house to one or more children but retain a "life estate," i.e., the right to possess the property during your lifetime. Upon your death, the title to the house passes automatically to the child or children to whom you deeded the house before; no additional deed is needed at that time. This can also be described as giving only a "remainder interest" in the house to your children.

Why would you want to do this? One reason is to reduce the amount of the gift, both for gift tax purposes (if you live in one of the gift tax states, discussed on page 56) and for Medicaid eligibility purposes. The other reason to transfer only a remainder interest is so that you can never be evicted from your own home. The interest of your children does not "vest" (i.e., they have no right to possession) until your death. So even if a child were sued or divorced during your lifetime, your interest in the house is protected.

How to Calculate the Gift

In order to calculate the amount of the gift you're making to the children when you sign a life estate deed, you first need two figures: your age and the value of your house. Next, look at the **"Life Estate Table (unisex)"** reproduced in the *Appendix* (see page 209), and find the "Remainder" number that corresponds with your age. Multiply that number by the value of your house to come up with the amount of the gift.

Example:

Assume you are age 65 and you sign a deed transferring your $250,000 house to your children, *but keeping a life estate interest in the house.* You consult the Table and see two figures to the right of age 65: .6797 and .3203. The first figure represents the value of your life estate (as a percentage of the value of 100% of the house) and the second figure represents the value of your gift of the remainder interest (again, equal to a percentage of the entire house). So in this case the remainder would be .3203, meaning that the gift to your children would be 32.03% of the current value of your house. If the house is worth $250,000 today, then signing a life estate deed would cause an immediate gift of $80,075 (32.03% x $250,000). Depending on the state you live in, that could cause a Medicaid penalty period of less than two years vs. more than five years had you transferred the entire value of the house to your children, instead.

Joint Interest vs. Remainder Interest Gift

Once you reach age 77, the gift of a remainder interest will exceed 50%, and the percentage increases as you get older. On the other hand, giving one child a joint interest on a deed will always be exactly 50% (in a state that does not permit deeding small percentages to a child with a right of survivorship). Thus, in such a state, adding a child to the deed will always result in a *smaller gift* than transferring a remainder interest, if you are age 77 or older.

That being said, you should also consider the creditor issues discussed above, which are avoided with a transfer of a remainder interest. Of course, if you plan to wait out the lookback period in any event, then the size of the gift is irrelevant (unless you live in one of the states that impose a gift tax (see page 56)).

Finally, the value of a life estate decreases with each passing year as the person on whose life the value is based (the "life tenant") gets older, whereas a fixed percentage interest in a house will never decrease in value (unless the value of the entire house decreases). This could be important if your state expands its definition of "estate" for estate recovery purposes to include the value of the life estate at the time of the Medicaid recipient's death (see page 157). Once the owner of a 50% joint interest passes age 77, the value of that joint interest will always be higher than that of a life estate, which continues to decrease as the life tenant ages.

Transfer to Trust, Keep Life Estate

An alternative to deeding a remainder interest to one or more children is that of deeding a remainder interest to a trust. Such a trust must be irrevocable and unamendable in order for this to work. Using a revocable "living" trust will not work, here, because the remainder interest owned by such a trust may still be considered owned by you when you apply for Medicaid.

The same gift calculations described above apply in this case, too. The biggest differences are (i) you can serve as the trustee of the trust, so if you need to sell or refinance the property, you won't have to get the signatures of your children first, and (ii) you can retain the ability to change the ultimate distribution of the house following your death, should you so desire (through exercise of a "power of appointment" clause included in the trust document).

Upon your death, the interest in your house will pass automatically to the trust, where it will be distributed as you have set forth in the trust document (or as you may have revised it by exercising your "power of appointment" given to you in the trust document).

Outright Transfer to Trust

You can also transfer the entire title to your house to an irrevocable trust. This will cause a period of disqualification based on the full value of the house on the date you sign the deed. Because of the home's value and the resulting lengthy penalty period, this technique will almost always require you to wait at least five years before applying for Medicaid. However, a clear advantage of this technique is that you will have absolutely no legal interest in the home at your death, thereby eliminating the possibility of estate recovery completely. You can also serve as the trustee of the trust, so that if you want to sell the house at any time, you would not need to obtain your children's signatures.

> NOTE: Although you are transferring the entire value of the house, the trust can be drafted so there will be no gift tax, which is important if you live in one of the gift tax states (page 56).

Ladybird Deed

In a number of states it is possible for you to transfer the home to someone else, typically your children, while retaining the legal right to sell or otherwise dispose of the house during your lifetime. This avoids probate at your death (and therefore avoids estate recovery, too, assuming the state does not have an expanded definition of "estate"). If you never sell or otherwise dispose of the house during your lifetime, then at your death ownership passes automatically to the individuals you deeded the house to, by operation of law, regardless of what your will says. Because you retain the power to sell or dispose of the house, signing the deed is not a gift; after all, you can essentially revoke the transfer at any time simply by signing a new deed transferring the house to someone else! This is quite similar in concept to a "beneficiary deed," which also allows you to list who will take title to your house if you still own it at the time of your death.

If this technique is available in your state, be sure to take advantage of this opportunity!

Purchase Life Estate in Child's Home

If it is possible for the parent to move into a child's home, this can be a wonderful method of protecting the parent's assets. The parent would sell his or her home and move in with the child. The child signs a deed transferring a percentage interest in the child's home equal to the value of the parent's life estate to the parent, and the parent transfers cash to the child in an amount equal to the value of that interest. *The parent must live in the child's house for at least one year after the deed is signed,* otherwise the Medicaid rules say that the purchase of the interest will be deemed to be a gift to the child of 100% of the amount the parent invested in the child's house.

Example:

Justin and his wife, Janice, recently purchased a home in an upscale part of town for $600,000. Janice's mom, Eunice, age 76, has been in declining health, needing assistance during the day. Her home and life savings together total $310,000. So Eunice sells her home and moves in with Justin and Janice, writing them a check for $302,646 in exchange for a life estate in their home. How did they come up with that amount? Based on the "**Life Estate Table (unisex)**" (see page 209), a person age 76 has a life estate valued at 50.441% and a remainder interest valued at 49.559%. Multiplying the value of the home ($600,000) by the value of Eunice's life estate (50.441%) gives you the value of the interest that Eunice is purchasing: $302,646.

If after a year Eunice has to move into a nursing home, her interest in her daughter's house will not be counted, since it is considered an interest in a personal residence, and such interest is almost always an excluded asset. Upon Eunice's death, her interest simply expires, leaving Justin and Janice once again as 100% owners of their home. Thus, there is nothing in Eunice's estate for the state Medicaid recovery unit to go after (assuming her state does not have an expanded definition of "estate"—see page 157).

Purchase Joint Interest in Child's Home

Because the life estate interest is fixed in percentage, it can be more advantageous for a parent to purchase a joint interest in a child's home and then move in.

Example:

Assume that Eunice (from the previous example) instead has $400,000 of assets and wants to move in with her daughter and son-in-law, Janice and Justin. If she purchases a life estate, as we saw, the most she can shelter is approximately $300,000. That would leave $100,000 ($400,000 - $300,000) exposed and Eunice would have too much money to qualify for Medicaid. Instead, she can purchase a 2/3 interest in the home ($400,000/$600,000) in exchange for her $400,000. The deed must specifically give Eunice a 2/3 interest in the house, and it must give a right of survivorship to the other owners of the house, so that upon her death her interest passes automatically to Justin and Janice, leaving nothing for the state Medicaid recovery unit to go after (assuming her state does not have an expanded definition of "estate"—see page 157).

NOTE: Not all states permit a right of survivorship among unequal joint owners of real estate.

Joint Interest vs. Life Estate Purchase in Child's Home

The reasons to consider *purchasing* a life estate interest vs. a joint interest in a child's home are similar to those discussed above when comparing the *gift* of a remainder interest and joint interest (see page 98).

Although the numbers may favor purchasing a life estate interest, one major factor that may or may not make a difference (depending on the parent's health) is that there is no one-year residency requirement for the joint purchase as there is with a life estate purchase. Theoretically, the parent could make the joint interest purchase, move in, and move out to a nursing home the next day, and the interest should still be a valid non-gift transaction. However, the longer the parent actually does reside in the child's home following the purchase, the better it looks to the Medicaid folks and the less trouble the parent will have.

Parent's Child Moves into the Home ("Caretaker Child")

See discussion of *Caretaker Child,* page 139.

Parent's Sibling Moves into the Home

See discussion of *Resident Sibling,* page 140.

Income Tax Basis of the Home

There are good reasons to make sure your home is included in your taxable estate (i.e., for estate tax purposes). Typically, there is no concern about actually owing estate taxes for anyone thinking about Medicaid eligibility. After all, your estate must exceed $2 million before you will be liable for estate tax (federal), and anyone with that much dough is usually not trying to become Medicaid eligible. However, it is important for *income tax* purposes for your house to be includible in your taxable estate.

There is a federal estate tax rule that says that as long as you retain a right to live in your house for the rest of your life, the house will be includible in your taxable estate for estate tax purposes. As a result, that causes the house to get a new income tax basis equal to the date of death value of the property, which will eliminate any capital gains upon a sale of the house immediately following your death. Your right to live in the house does not even have to be in writing; it is enough if there was an implied agreement that you could continue to live there for the rest of your life.

Example:

If you bought your house in 1965 for $50,000 (the *basis*) and at your death it's worth $350,000, there's a capital gain of $300,000. If the tax is at the 15% rate, that's a tax of $45,000! However, if the house is included in your taxable estate, it gets a new income tax basis of $350,000. So if your family sells the house right after your death, they would pay zero capital gains taxes, saving $45,000.

ANNUITIES

Annuities have become one of the most popular investments in recent years.

> In its most basic form, a person transfers money to an insurance company in exchange for the company's contractual agreement to invest that money and pay it back to the owner with interest over an agreed-upon period of time. The reasons for annuities' popularity are (i) the investment inside the annuity grows on a tax-deferred basis, (ii) the investment can have a "guaranteed minimum" return of capital so that your annuity cannot drop below the amount of your initial investment, and (iii) they often contain a life insurance component.

In the following discussion, it is important to understand the following terms:

- The "**owner**" of an annuity is the person who has the right to change the beneficiary designation of the annuity.

- The "**annuitant**" is the person on whose life expectancy the payments of the annuity are based.

- The "**beneficiary**" is the person or group of persons who receive the annuity payments upon the death of the annuitant. With a Medicaid annuity, beneficiaries only receive such payments *if* there is a "guarantee period" and the annuitant dies before the end of his life expectancy. Otherwise, the payments stop upon the death of the annuitant.

- The "**guarantee period**" is the length of time the annuity payments must be made, whether or not the annuitant survives the entire period. Normally, an annuity would automatically terminate upon the death of the annuitant. However, that could be risky, because you never know how long a person will live. For example, what if the annuitant has a life expectancy of, say, 20 years but dies unexpectedly in year 2? If the annuity payments stop at the death of the annuitant, then most of the money used to purchase that annuity is lost. Instead, had the annuity been purchased with a

20-year guarantee period, then even if the annuitant died in year 2, payments would continue for the remaining 18 years, to the beneficiaries. Because the company that sells the annuity has greater exposure with an annuity with a guarantee period, the annuity payments will necessarily be lower for the same amount of money invested in the annuity.

The type of annuity that is most common is the "deferred variable annuity." This type of annuity does not have a specific amount that pays out on a regular basis, and it may simply sit there, growing over time, based on market conditions. This is called the "accumulation phase." At some point, all annuities must make payments, either to the owner, the annuitant, or one or more beneficiaries (after the death of the annuitant); that's called the "annuitization" or "payout" phase. If the annuity starts to pay back the investor as soon as it is purchased, then it is called an "immediate" annuity.

For Medicaid planning, there is a wonderful way to convert countable assets to non-countable: purchase a FIXED, IMMEDIATE ANNUITY. Such an annuity is sometimes referred to as a **"Medicaid Annuity" or "Medicaid-friendly Annuity."**

Because the payments are "fixed," you will receive a check for the same amount every month, regardless of the performance of the stock market. (A "variable" annuity is invested in the stock market, so that your annuity payments can go up or down, depending on the performance of your investment.) However, there is no opportunity to withdraw the principal of the annuity: once you purchase the annuity, all you will ever receive back is a series of regular equal payments, for the rest of the annuity term, which could be for a fixed number of years or over the remainder of your life.

Another type of annuity may start out as a deferred annuity (i.e., payments back to the owner have not yet started) and then convert to an immediate, fixed annuity upon the occurrence of some defined event, such as entering a nursing home. This type may also be called a "Medicaid-friendly Annuity."

Why Annuities Work in Medicaid Planning

The main reason annuities are such a powerful Medicaid planning technique is that once you purchase a "Medicaid annuity," it is no longer a countable asset. Instead, the payments back to the owner are countable solely as payments of income. In effect, you can take $100,000 and buy the right kind of annuity, and suddenly that entire $100,000 has "disappeared" for Medicaid eligibility purposes! However, there are certain rules that must be followed if you want this to work.

General Requirements

The annuity must be fixed, immediate, irrevocable, and non-transferable.

"Fixed" means that the regularly occurring payments of the annuity amount must always be the same, and they must not be dependent on the stock market's performance, as would be the case with a variable annuity.

"Immediate" means that the payments back to the owner must start immediately following the purchase of the annuity, unlike the more common "deferred" annuity which may not pay anything back to the owner for a number of years.

"Irrevocable" means that once you sign the contract to purchase the annuity, you can neither change its terms nor get your money back.

"Non-transferable" means that you cannot transfer or assign the ownership of the annuity to anyone. You cannot sell it. After all, if you could sell the annuity, then the state Medicaid department could logically demand that you do so, and then apply the proceeds to your nursing home bill. But if the annuity cannot be sold, then it has no value as an asset, other than the stream of income that it pays to you.

By the way, an "SPIA" is insurance industry-speak for Single Premium Immediate Annuity, which is the only kind acceptable for Medicaid purposes.

NOTE: Several states have taken the position recently that even though the annuity contract states that it cannot be sold, it still must be valued as a "countable" asset if there are businesses that would sign a contract with the owner of the annuity, exchanging a lump sum payment for an unsecured promise by the owner to pay over each annuity payment as it is received. Although some of the states have lost court cases in this area, it is clearly an evolving area that requires an experienced elder law attorney who is aware of the cases and trends in your own state, to assist you with Medicaid annuity purchases.

Payback to State

Under the federal Deficit Reduction Act of 2005 (as amended on 12/20/06), effective for all Medicaid annuities issued on or after Feb. 8, 2006, in order to prevent having the purchase of a Medicaid annuity treated as a gift, the state must be named as the successor beneficiary of the annuity payments after the death of the "institutionalized individual," i.e., the person in the nursing home. This is to ensure that the state will be reimbursed out of the remaining annuity payments (if any) for any Medicaid payments it made on behalf of such person. However, if there is a spouse or a minor or disabled child who is named as the successor beneficiary, then the state may be named as second successor after such person(s). Note, however, that the above requirements do not apply if the annuity is an Individual Retirement Annuity or purchased with proceeds from an IRA, SEP, SIMPLE, or Roth IRA.

Single Person Annuity Purchase

Age

Some annuity companies will not issue an annuity based on an annuitant who is over age 85, but others will go as high as 90 or beyond.

Amount

An annuity may be purchased for a single (unmarried) individual in any amount.

Term

If the term of the annuity is based on a life expectancy greater than that of the annuitant, then some portion of the purchase price will be considered a gift, for Medicaid purposes.

///   **Let's take a look at an example.**

For the rest of this section we are going to follow John, age 65 and unmarried, who because of unfortunate health problems is facing nursing home care for an indefinite period. In order to shelter a portion of his assets, he is considering purchasing a Medicaid annuity. Since he is moving into the nursing home immediately, it's important to him that he does not incur any penalty period.

First, John should look up his life expectancy on the federally published table (see **Annuity (Life Expectancy) Table**, page 207). According to this table, a male age 65 has a life expectancy of 16.05 years. Therefore, so long as John purchases an annuity based on his life expectancy, or based on a guaranteed series of equal payments that cannot exceed his life expectancy of 16 years (the "guarantee period"), there will be no gift for Medicaid purposes. As a result, the full cost of the annuity will be /// sheltered and deemed a non-countable asset.

Payments

Each payment to John will be deemed a payment of income in the month received. If any portion of the payment is not spent within the month it is received, such portion will be counted as part of John's assets as of the first day of the following month. If John is in the nursing home at the time the annuity is in effect, then (after deducting some permitted allowances—see page 148) he must pay the entire amount of each payment to the nursing home.

How to Estimate the Monthly Payments

A good estimate of the monthly annuity payments a Medicaid applicant will receive following his or her purchase may be found at this website: http://www.immediateannuities.com/

Here's how to use this for Medicaid planning purposes:

1) Select the state where the Medicaid applicant lives (box 1). Let's assume John lives in Colorado.

2) Select the age of the Medicaid applicant (box 2) We know John is age 65.
3) Select the gender of the Medicaid applicant (box 3)
4) Ignore the spouse options (boxes 4 and 5)
5) Enter the amount you wish to protect in the box that says "Enter the Dollar Amount you have to invest ('Deposit')" Let's assume John wishes to protect $100,000.
6) Click the Calculate button.
7) Find the Estimated Monthly Income in the top section. Look for the guarantee period closest to the Medicaid Table life expectancy. So for John, a male age 65, the life expectancy is 16.05 years (which you got from the Table in the Appendix), so we use the "Single Lifetime Income with Up to 15 Years Guaranteed to Your Beneficiary ("15CC")".
8) Summary: For a male, 65, in Colorado, investing $100,000, the monthly annuity check would be approximately $656.

HERE'S AN ALTERNATE WEBSITE FOR A SECOND OPINION:

http://www.brkdirect.com/spia/EZQUOTE.ASP

Here's how to use this for Medicaid planning purposes:

1) Click Male or Female (this is for the potential Medicaid applicant whose money will be used to purchase the annuity)
2) Enter the person's birth date
3) Skip the Joint Annuitant section (this is only for married couples)
4) Click "Investment" and enter the amount of money you plan to use to buy the annuity, in the box on the right.
5) Set "Periodicity" to "Monthly" (this means your family member will be getting a monthly check)
6) Enter the proposed date you want this to start, such as the first day of next month.
7) Under "Payment Options" click "Guaranteed Minimum Payment" and enter the number of months of their life expectancy: Multiply the number of years of the person's life expectancy (which you got from the Table in the Appendix) x 12.
8) Select your state
9) Click the box "Periodic Benefit".

10) After a few seconds, you will see your results in the green box under your entry section (you may have to scroll down a little). Look for the monthly payment figure.

For a more accurate quote, you will need to contact an agent that sells these types of Medicaid annuities. See the Resources list in the *Appendix* for some suggestions.

Normal Life Expectancy

Problem. If John must turn over every annuity payment to the nursing home, and if the payments must stop upon John's death, at first blush it appears that there is no benefit to this type of annuity: At John's death, the annuity payments stop, and no part of the money ever gets to his other family members.

Shorter Than Normal Life Expectancy

Benefit. If John's annuity had a guarantee period equal to his life expectancy of 16 years, and John dies after, say, 5 years, then the annuity does not stop at his death, but must continue for the remainder of the guarantee period, i.e., 11 more years. Assume that the monthly payments will be $650 per month. So if John invested $100,000 in the annuity and turned over every payment he received to the nursing home ($650 per month x 60 months), and died after 5 years, his family will receive the balance of the monthly payments for the next 11 years: $650 x 12 months x 11 years = $85,800.

(NOTE: In most cases the family cannot terminate the annuity and cash it in; they must simply wait and receive each annuity payment according to the same payment schedule that was in effect while John was alive. There are only a few companies that will allow the beneficiaries to cash out; if that is something John wants, then he will have to accept slightly reduced monthly payments in exchange for this option.)

However, if John had qualified for Medicaid coverage, upon his death the annuity payments must go to the state, up to the amount of Medicaid payments it made on John's behalf. So the benefit to his family would have to be reduced accordingly.

If the state must be paid back, does it still make sense to purchase an annuity? It might, *if* certain conditions exist. By qualifying the annuity owner for

Medicaid, the payments to the nursing home are reduced. This "stretches out" the benefit of the annuity and reduces the amount of total cost to the family.

⫻ Example:

John, age 65, invests $100,000 in an annuity that will pay him $650 per month, so that he can qualify for Medicaid to pay his nursing home expenses. His other income is Social Security of $800 per month. Each month both his Social Security and annuity payment must be turned over to the nursing home; Medicaid pays the balance of the bill. If the "Medicaid reimbursement rate" for John's nursing home is $3,500 per month, then each month the state is paying the nursing home $3,500 - $800 - $650 = $2,050. If John dies after 5 years, this adds up to 60 months x $2,050 = $123,000. The state must first be satisfied out of the remaining annuity payments (equal to $85,800), leaving a balance owed to the state of $37,200 (assume there is estate recovery against John's home). Total cost to John and his estate: $137,200 ($100,000 annuity investment + $37,200 of estate recovery).

If John does not purchase the annuity he will have to spend down his $100,000 paying the nursing home at the "private pay" rate, of, say $5,000 per month. His monthly out-of-pocket costs would be $5,000 - $800 (Social Security) = $4,200. Thus his $100,000 will be depleted after 24 months. At that point he will qualify for Medicaid. Assuming, again, that John dies after 5 years, Medicaid will cover him for the next 36 months, until his death, at a cost of $97,200 ($3,500 - $800 = $2,700 x 36). Again, assume there is estate recovery against John's home for this amount. Total cost to John and his estate: $197,200 ($100,000 assets + $97,200 of estate recovery).

As you can see, by purchasing the annuity, even though no part of that annuity money will ever be paid to other family members, John's family actually *saves $60,000* because the estate recovery bill has been reduced.

That being said, **if John had no other assets in his name at the time of his death, then it would make no difference whether he purchases the annuity or not**, since in either case upon his death his "assets" are limited to the annuity. So either he spends the $100,000 and then qualifies for Medicaid or he purchases an annuity, qualifies for Medicaid sooner, but then lives long enough to run up a bill owed to the state at least equal to the value of the remaining annuity payments. In either case, his family receives nothing at his death.

If John had died after only one year, however, then the reduction in the nursing home costs by paying the Medicaid rate, as opposed to the private pay rate, would indeed have saved the family money, even assuming full repayment to the state. After all, it saved him $1,500 per month. The breakeven point is as follows: Once the amount owed to the state equals or exceeds the value of the remaining annuity payments, there is no longer any benefit to the annuity.

BOTTOM LINE FOR UNMARRIED INDIVIDUALS: In most cases, unless the potential Medicaid applicant (i) has a *very* short life expectancy (such that the amount of Medicaid benefits subject to state payback at the applicant's death is less than the value of the remaining annuity payments) *or* (ii) owns a home that might be subject to estate recovery for the balance owed to the state after subtracting the value of the remaining annuity payments, it does not make economic sense to purchase a Medicaid annuity for a single individual if state rules will require payback. (Notwithstanding the above, often a combination of a gift and an annuity will make sense where purchase of an annuity alone will not. See page 133.)

Married Couple Annuity Purchase

With a married couple you can either base the annuity period on the age of the spouse in the nursing home or on that of the Community Spouse. However, under the new law enacted in 2006 (the DRA), as amended in December 2006 by the Tax Relief and Health Care Act of 2006, the state must be named as a beneficiary of the annuity, so that it can be reimbursed for any Medicaid benefits it paid on behalf of the "institutionalized individual."

So if the nursing home spouse purchases an annuity and dies, the full amount of Medicaid payments the state made on that spouse's behalf must be paid back out of the remaining annuity payments, to the extent of their value (although if there is a surviving spouse or a minor or disabled child named as successor beneficiary, the state will have to wait until the death of such person(s) to collect on this debt (see page 109)). This cannot necessarily be avoided by having the Community Spouse purchase the annuity and receive the annuity payments, since the amount of Medicaid payments made on behalf of the nursing home spouse must *still* be paid back—out of the annuity—upon the death of the Community Spouse.

However, if the annuity payments have stopped during the lifetime of the Community Spouse, then there will be no remainder available at the death of the Community Spouse from which to repay the state.

Thus, it will normally make the most sense to purchase as short an annuity as possible, if the Community Spouse is going to be the recipient of the annuity payments.

Note that if the Community Spouse is the owner of the annuity and is receiving monthly payments, if the Community Spouse him- or herself winds up in the nursing home at some point in the future, the state rules may require that the beneficiary designation name the state so it can be reimbursed for any Medicaid benefits it paid on behalf of the "institutionalized individual," which is now the Community Spouse. If the state was only named the beneficiary as to payments it made on behalf of the *nursing home spouse* and not the Community Spouse, it may require that the beneficiary designation be changed. The literal language of the new federal amendment seems to indicate that the state need only be repaid for the costs of the person who is the "institutionalized individual" *at the time of the annuity purchase.* By definition, the Community Spouse is never an "institutionalized individual" at the time of the annuity purchase. However, since this is a new law and there are no state regulations interpreting this, yet, you will need to check your own state's regulations before you actually purchase a Medicaid annuity for a married person.

Another reason to have the annuity payments made to the Community Spouse is so that the payments are not "wasted" by having them paid to the nursing home, as they must be with an unmarried person's annuity. Since all of the annuity payments are made to the Community Spouse, and the income of the Community Spouse never has to be transferred to the nursing home spouse, this means that

100% of the annuity money can essentially be retained by the family unit, while permitting the nursing home spouse immediately to qualify for Medicaid.

The only consideration is that the annuity period may not exceed the life expectancy of the annuitant spouse (such as the Community Spouse) without causing a gift. This is the same rule as applies to an annuity purchased for a single individual, discussed above.

In some states, if the annuity payment to the Community Spouse causes the income of that spouse to exceed the MMMNA, then the portion of the annuity that causes such excess will be considered a gift (to the named beneficiaries of the annuity, which is typically the children). This would apply only to the extent that the gifted amount causes the CSRA to exceed the maximum (currently $101,640), but typically a Medicaid annuity would not be purchased unless there *were* excess assets: after all, the main purpose of buying the annuity was to convert those excess countable assets into a non-countable annuity.

In such a state, the lower the income of both spouses, the greater the amount of the annuity that can be purchased without creating a gift that causes a penalty period. Unfortunately, smaller monthly payments means a longer annuity period, which is the opposite of what you normally would want: as discussed above, the shorter the annuity payout period, the less chance the state will ever get paid back for the Medicaid payments it made on behalf of the nursing home spouse. Remember, it's only the annuity payments continuing after the Community Spouse's death that the state can tap into for repayment.

Effect on Community Spouse's Income

The Community Spouse is entitled to a minimum amount of income per month, under federal law. Until July 1, 2007, this amount—known as the Minimum Monthly Maintenance Needs Allowance ('MMMNA")—is $1,650.If the Community Spouse's income (from Social Security, pensions, etc.) is less than this amount, then the Community Spouse is entitled to shift the amount necessary to bring the Community Spouse up to this amount, from the income of the nursing home spouse. (See detailed discussion of these rules beginning on page 26.)

So *if the Community Spouse's income is less than the MMMNA*, and that income is suddenly increased following the purchase of a Medicaid annuity, then that can reduce or eliminate the ability to shift income from the nursing home spouse to the Community Spouse. As a result, more of the couple's joint income will be "wasted" in paying for nursing home care that Medicaid otherwise would have paid for. This result must be considered and brought into any calculation of the benefits of having the Community Spouse purchase a Medicaid annuity.

Notwithstanding the above, an annuity may still be worth purchasing because it can continue after the death of the nursing home spouse. If the Community Spouse were relying on the income of the nursing home spouse as a supplement, that income will typically end upon the death of the nursing home spouse. The income from the annuity, however, will almost always continue for the lifetime of the Community Spouse. So it is a more reliable, long-term benefit, all other things being equal.

Example:

Martha lives in the community while her husband, Daniel, is in the nursing home. They own a home and have excess countable assets of $200,000. Martha's only income is $975 of Social Security; Daniel's income is $1,500 from a pension and Social Security. Under the MMMNA rules discussed above, Martha is entitled to have *at least* $1,650 of income per month. Since her income is less than that, she would be entitled to shift some of her husband's income over to her to bring her income up to $1,650. Thus, she's entitled to $675 of Daniel's income; he must pay the rest of his income to the nursing home, and once he's on Medicaid, it will pick up the balance of his nursing home bill.

However, this couple won't qualify for Medicaid because they have approximately $100,000 of excess assets. So Martha decides to convert the extra $100,000 to a Medicaid annuity. At age 71 she can purchase an annuity that does not exceed her table life expectancy of 14.65 years. This annuity will generate approximately $675 of additional income for Martha. Since her income from Social Security is $975, the annuity payments will increase her income to $1,650 per month. As a result, she will not be entitled to shift any of Daniel's income to herself. In a way, that extra $675 of Daniel's income she *could* have shifted to herself is "wasted," in that now it must be paid to the nursing home, where all it will accomplish is a reduction of what Medicaid has to pay. However, this plan still makes sense, because it permits Daniel to qualify for Medicaid immediately. In addition, upon Daniel's death, his pension and Social Security will terminate, and if that $100,000 excess had been spent on his nursing home care instead of used to purchase the annuity, Martha's income would be at $975 and not $1,650, for the rest of her life.

Effect on Community Spouse's Assets (CSRA)

If the total income of *both* spouses is less than the MMMNA, having income from a Medicaid annuity paid to the Community Spouse could prevent the ability to protect additional assets under the theory that such assets would be needed to generate additional income (by a Fair Hearing to increase the CSRA, as discussed on page 45). Indeed, if the couple's income is low enough—or if the MMMNA can be increased enough—it may be possible for the Community Spouse to protect sufficient additional assets this way without needing to purchase an annuity at all.

Deciding on the Length of the Annuity Term

There are competing goals in deciding the length of the annuity term. To minimize the income of the Community Spouse, you want the annuity to be for as long a period of time as possible without causing it to be a gift, i.e., up to the full "table" life expectancy of the Community Spouse. That's because the longer the term, the lower each monthly payment to the Community Spouse. And the lower the Community Spouse's income, the more income that can be shifted from the nursing home spouse. Indeed, if after each annuity payment the total income of both spouses is still below the MMMNA, additional assets can be sheltered as part of the CSRA (thereby reducing the amount of the annuity needed). However, the longer the annuity term the greater the possibility that the Community Spouse will die before receiving all of the annuity payments. As discussed above, that could expose those payments to a repayment claim of the state.

In order to figure out what to do, first look at the income of the Community Spouse (Social Security plus pensions, etc.). If it's *above* the MMMNA (and remember, that can be adjusted above the minimum, in certain cases), then you might as well get as short an annuity as you can, since in that situation there's no way to shift additional income or assets to the Community Spouse. If the Community Spouse's income is *below* the MMMNA, then you have to look at the amount of income or assets that can be shifted and balance that against the life expectancy of the Community Spouse: The longer the Community Spouse is expected to live (relative to his or her "table" life expectancy), the more sense it makes to get a longer-term annuity. That will permit shifting income (and possibly assets, too) without too much risk that the Community Spouse will die before receiving most or all of the annuity payments. (If the payment period is for the longer of a guaranteed term of years *or* the life of the Community Spouse, then it only matters if the Community Spouse dies before the end of the guarantee period; after that, whether or not the Community Spouse has actually lived to his or her full life expectancy is irrelevant, because the payments will end at the Community Spouse's death, leaving nothing for repayment to the state.)

Calculating the Gift

If an annuity is purchased with a guarantee period longer than the life expectancy of the annuitant, then the amount of money attributable to the excess payments is deemed a gift. So if your life expectancy is 15 years, and you purchase a Medicaid annuity with a guarantee period of 20 years, then the gift is equal to the difference between the cost of an annuity with a 15-year guarantee period and total cost of the purchased annuity. As a general rule, it makes more sense simply to make a current outright gift of that excess amount rather than purchase a longer annuity, because the annuity purchase incurs a significant commission cost, ties up the money inside the annuity, and subjects an additional amount to possible state payback.

Annuity Purchase by the Community Spouse

Consider having the Community Spouse purchase a large annuity at least five years prior to the necessity of the other spouse applying for Medicaid. Since the purchase will involve a gift (see above), once the five-year lookback period has passed, the transfer will be ignored. And, since the annuity payments to the Community Spouse are not attributable to the nursing home spouse, the Community Spouse will essentially get the benefit of the entire amount of money used to purchase the annuity. In other words, even though it may be deemed a gift for Medicaid eligibility purposes, in reality, the purchasing spouse is retaining all the payments of income (i.e., the annuity payments) back to him- or herself.

Although there is no theoretical limit on the amount of assets that can be sheltered this way, there is a practical limit. For example, if a couple has $500,000 of excess resources and the healthy spouse purchases a Medicaid annuity payable to himself five years in advance of his wife applying for Medicaid, it's true that, by the time of the Medicaid application, the $500,000 annuity will be ignored, since it was purchased outside of the five-year lookback period. However, the monthly annuity payment may be so large that the Community Spouse does not spend it all each month, so that by the time the wife applies for Medicaid, some of those payments have accumulated, causing the couple to have excess resources, again. As a result, the wife will not be eligible for Medicaid until those excess resources are spent down or otherwise disposed of.

What if the couple is concerned that the less-healthy spouse may need to enter a nursing home prior to the expiration of the five-year period, following the annuity purchase? In that case, the couple should consider immediately purchasing long-term care insurance for the less-healthy spouse, if at all possible. It is a good way to hedge one's bets, particularly when health is still good currently, but you are doing some long-term planning. If the health of the ill spouse precludes purchasing a long-term care insurance policy, then the couple should be sure to retain sufficient assets in addition to the CSRA to cover the anticipated cost of the nursing home, for the period prior to the expiration of the five-year lookback period. You don't want to retain *too* many assets, however, in case it turns out that the ill spouse didn't need nursing home care as soon as you thought, leaving you with excess assets at the end of the lookback period. As you can see, this involves guessing how long it may be before the less healthy spouse may need to move to a nursing home, so you need to consider all the different possible scenarios when deciding how much to set aside.

Recent Developments

Although specifically permitted under federal law, the so-called "Medicaid annuity" discussed above allows so much money to be converted from countable to non-countable that a number of states have passed laws restricting their use. One type of restriction has already been discussed, that of limiting the amount of the annuity for a Community Spouse to that necessary to increase the Community Spouse's income to the MMMNA. Other states have attempted to restrict their use by requiring that even non-transferable annuities must be valued as if they could be sold on the open market. Once again, it is absolutely necessary to have a local elder law attorney discuss this with you, so that you will know whether or not these techniques are available in your state.

IRAs and Converting to an Annuity

Any withdrawal from an IRA or qualified retirement plan (401(k), 403(b), etc.) will normally be taxed as part of the ordinary income of the IRA owner in the year of withdrawal, unless it can be annuitized (see below). For a single individual applying for Medicaid, the IRA or other qualified retirement plan will have to be liquidated, unless it can be annuitized (see below). For married couples, if the nursing home spouse has an IRA, then it will probably have to be completely withdrawn in order to transfer the money into the Community Spouse's name. If the IRA is so large that part of it will be taxed in a higher bracket than the rest of the Medicaid applicant's assets, then try to spread the withdrawals out over more than one calendar year, so as to reduce the overall tax bill. If you need to reduce the Medicaid applicant's assets in as short a time period as possible, then deferring the total withdrawal of the IRA may not make sense: you will probably wind up paying more to the nursing home for the extra months the Medicaid applicant is disqualified from Medicaid than you'll save in income taxes from the deferral into a second calendar year. (An exception is the Roth IRA: since this was taxed when the IRA converted to the Roth IRA, there is no tax upon withdrawal.)

A little-known option is that of converting an IRA into a "Medicaid annuity" (see page 107). It is usually possible to convert an IRA into an annuity without having to withdraw the entire amount of the IRA. You will need to discuss this with your financial advisor or IRA administrator, who probably will not be familiar with Medicaid annuity planning. If so, you should show them the discussion in this book and make sure they also check with an experienced elder law attorney. The main advantage of this conversion is that the IRA will not have to be withdrawn all at once, saving you thousands of dollars in income tax, *and* you avoid the requirement that the state be named as the beneficiary of the annuity.

The annuity must be paid to the IRA owner and must be based on the owner's life expectancy, as well. To decide if the IRA should be annuitized or simply withdrawn requires an analysis of the Medicaid annuity rules in the context of the Medicaid applicant's entire financial and health situation. See page 109 for further discussion of annuity planning.

Private Annuities

A "private annuity" is simply an annuity arrangement between family members, as opposed to a commercial annuity involving an insurance company. The big advantage with a private annuity is that if the family member on whose life the annuity payments are based dies early, it means that the family will keep all the payments that did not have to be made. With a commercial annuity, if the person receiving the annuity payments dies earlier than expected, then—depending on the type of annuity you purchased—the payments stop and the insurance company profits at the family's expense.

Since not all states allow the use of a private annuity, be sure to check before you set one of these up among family members.

Balloon Payment

With an unmarried Medicaid recipient, every payment of the annuity must go either to the nursing home or to allowable medical expenses, reducing what Medicaid would otherwise have paid. So for a Medicaid recipient with no other assets, it really does not benefit the family at all unless the recipient dies before his or her "table" life expectancy, i.e., the number of years the Medicaid recipient is "expected" to live based on the federally mandated life expectancy tables used for these purposes. As a result, the smaller the monthly payments, the more will be available to go to family members upon the nursing home resident's death.

One way to achieve this is to reduce the monthly payments to a very low amount, with the difference being added to a single large final payment just before the expiration of the nursing home resident's life expectancy. Because the payment amount "balloons" in size for that final payment, this is known as a "balloon payment" annuity. However, the Deficit Reduction Act passed in 2006 disqualifies any annuity contract that includes a "balloon" payment option, so this technique is only useful in rare circumstances.

Chapter 13

PROMISSORY NOTES

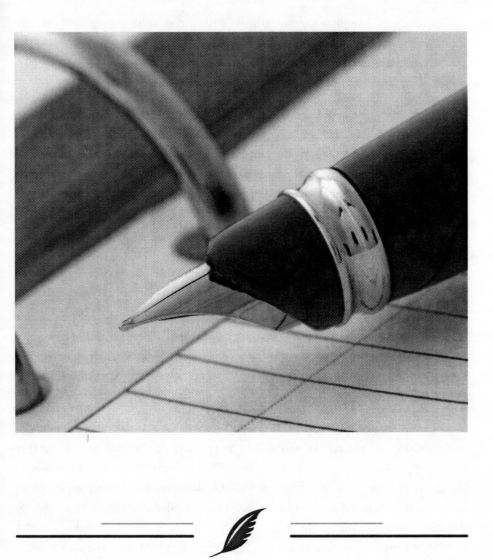

A "promissory note" or "note" is simply an IOU. For Medicaid planning purposes, a properly structured promissory note is ignored, meaning that you can make money disappear by lending it to someone else!

The promissory note must meet the following requirements for this to work:

1) It cannot require payments over a period of time longer than the life expectancy of the lender;
2) All payments must be equal in amount; and
3) The note cannot be cancelable upon the lender's death.

In order to avoid having the loan from the person in the nursing home counted as a gift of the entire amount loaned, there must be a promissory note documenting the loan. It should set out the names of the lender and the borrower, the amount of the loan, the term of the loan (i.e., how long until the loan must be completely repaid), the amount of each payment back to the lender, the amount of interest charged (if any), etc.

Length of Payment Term

If the lender is to be the family member in the nursing home, then the smaller each payment back to the lender, the better. After all, the payment will simply be applied to the nursing home bill and only serve to reduce what Medicaid pays the nursing home. In other words, it won't benefit the family member in the nursing home.

You might be tempted to stretch out the payments over, say, a 40-year period, even if the family member in the nursing home is 85. After all, the greater the number of payments, the smaller each payment will be. However, to avoid making a gift that will cause the family member to be disqualified from receiving Medicaid for a period of time, the term of the loan cannot exceed the life expectancy of the lender at the time the loan is made. To find the correct life expectancy, you use the same table used for annuity purchases (see **Annuity (Life Expectancy) Table**, page 207).

Example:

Lulu resides in a nursing home and has $51,000 in her bank account and no other assets. To qualify for Medicaid, Lulu decides to lend $50,000 to her son, so she can then immediately apply for Medicaid. Because Lulu is age 70, you would look at the Annuity (Life Expectancy) Tables for Female Life Expectancy, age 70. The table indicates that her life expectancy is 15.35 years. This means that the loan must be repaid within this time period. Converting this to months, it means that the loan cannot exceed a total of 184.2 months. To be conservative, always round down to the nearest whole month.

Equal Payments

Once you know how long the loan will last (i.e., its "term"), it's a simple matter to determine the amount of each monthly payment: divide the amount of the loan by the number of months of the term.

Example:

Lulu's life expectancy is 184 months, so divide the amount of the loan—$50,000—by 184, to get $271.74. This figure represents the amount that the lender must pay to Lulu each month, for the term of the loan: 184 months. (This assumes no interest is charged.)

Other Important Clauses of the Note

- **NON-CANCELABLE:** The note must prohibit cancellation upon the death of the lender.

- **NAME A BENEFICIARY:** If the laws of your state permit it, and recovery is only permitted against the probate estate, then the note itself should name a successor to whom the payments will be made upon the death of the lender. This will avoid having the note payments flow through the probate estate of the lender, thereby subjecting them to estate recovery.

  If your state does not permit this, the remaining payments must be made to the estate of the lender, where they will be subject to a recovery claim by the state (see page 155). If your state has adopted the "expanded" definition of "estate" (see page 157), then this will not matter, since the unpaid balance of the note will be subject to estate recovery in either case.

- **NON-ASSIGNABLE:** The note must state that it cannot be pledged, canceled, or assigned by the lender. If the note cannot be sold, transferred or pledged as collateral for a loan, then its only value is as a stream of income, *not* as an asset, and the state cannot claim otherwise.

Interest Rate Charged

There is no requirement that a certain amount of interest be charged for the loan. As a general rule, it is probably best not to charge *any* interest. That reduces the amount of each payment back to the lender (the parent) and simplifies the calculations, too.

However, if less interest is charged than what the federal government says is the going rate for a loan of the type you've signed then there are income tax consequences. The difference between the interest you charged—if any—and the amount the government says is the going rate at the time of your loan, is known as "foregone" interest.

In addition, the foregone interest for each year is treated as a *taxable gift* from the lender to the borrower. However, no actual out-of-pocket federal gift tax will have to be paid by the lender unless the total amount of lifetime gifts made by the lender exceeds $1,000,000! (If the lender happens to live in Connecticut, Louisiana, North Carolina, or Tennessee, there is a state gift tax that may apply here, in addition to the federal gift tax (see page 56). Be sure to consult your attorney about the possible impact of this state gift tax on the technique discussed in this section.)

Thus, if no interest is being paid to the lender, there are two results: (i) there is an "imputed" interest payment to the lender from the borrower, and (ii) there is a deemed *gift* of the imputed interest from the lender *to* the borrower, as if made on the last day of each calendar year. Luckily, there are monetary loan limits under which the imputed interest is treated as zero. These can be very complex to calculate.

BOTTOM LINE: It's best to consult an accountant to help you figure out the imputed income, to avoid getting in trouble with the IRS!

NO INTEREST LOAN

Recent Developments

Some states have begun to institute regulations that characterize promissory notes as countable resources, even if they meet the requirements on page 124. Although this seems directly to contradict the federal statute, it points out once again the hazards of trying to do these techniques on your own, without the advice of an experienced and up-to-date elder law attorney.

Chapter 14

TRANSFER (GIFT) STRATEGIES

The "Half-A-Loaf" Method

A very popular method of spending down excess resources is called the "half-a-loaf" method. Essentially, it works like this: You give away approximately half of your countable assets, which results in a penalty period. However, you can now use the other half to pay for your living expenses or nursing home costs during this period. At the end of the penalty period, you should just run out of money, so that now you can apply for and qualify for Medicaid coverage.

Example:

Roland is about to enter a nursing home. He has $102,000 in the bank and his only income is Social Security of $1,000 per month. The nursing home costs $6,000 per month, meaning that it's reducing his bank account by $5,000 per month ($6,000 total cost - $1,000 income). At the rate of $5,000 a month, if Roland does no planning, he will have spent $100,000 in 20 months, leaving him with only $2,000. At that point, he will be able to qualify for Medicaid coverage of his nursing home expenses.

But Roland will have spent all his money. Instead, Roland gives away all of his money to his children ($100,000), except for the $2,000 exclusion amount. Assuming the state penalty divisor is $5,000, this will result in a penalty period of 20 months. In other words, he cannot qualify for Medicaid coverage for 20 months after the date he made this gift. Who will pay the nursing home during this time? Unfortunately, his children, recipients of the gift, will have to use the very money Roland just gave them, to pay the nursing home for the penalty period. At the end of the 20 months, Roland will be past the penalty period, and since he will only have $2,000, he will then qualify for Medicaid. But it took the full $100,000 of his money, leaving his children with nothing.

As you can see, **there is no benefit to Roland giving away all his money to his children,** because they'll just have to turn around and use that money to pay for his nursing home care during the resulting penalty period.

The "half-a-loaf" method is a vast improvement, saving him approximately half of his money. Here's how it works:

Roland gives his children not $100,000, but *half* that amount, or $50,000. That results in a 10-month penalty period ($50,000 ÷ $5,000 = 10). Roland still has $52,000 left, so he simply pays the nursing home himself, for the 10-month period. At the end of the 10 months, the penalty period expires, and Roland is down to just $2,000. At that point, he can immediately apply for Medicaid coverage and based on his assets and income, he should qualify. Result? He only had to wait 10 months, not 20, and his children have the $50,000 that Roland gave them.

Amount saved: $50,000.

Unfortunately, the numbers almost never work out as cleanly as the above. Accordingly, there is a formula you can use to calculate the proper amount to give away. In the following, "income" includes only regularly occurring income such as Social Security, pension, Railroad Retirement, etc. It does *not* include interest and dividends from the bank accounts or other investments of the person applying for Medicaid.

THE HALF-A-LOAF FORMULA
[Countable assets ÷ (A + B) = # of months penalty] x B = amount to transfer
Explanation of Formula:
Countable assets ÷ (net monthly expenses + state penalty divisor) = number of months penalty.
Multiply that number by the state penalty divisor = amount to transfer.

Start with the **total amount of countable assets.** For a single person, this is all countable assets minus $2,000. For a married couple, subtract the amount the nursing home spouse can retain ($2,000) and also subtract the Community Spouse's CSRA ($101,640 in many states, or 50% of the total countable assets of both spouses up to a maximum of $101,640, in the other states; if the total assets are $20,328 or less, the Community Spouse can keep it all, even in those states that divide by 2).

Calculate the **net monthly expenses ("A")** of (i) single person (living expenses + nursing home cost - total income) or (ii) married couple (living expenses of Community Spouse + nursing home cost - total income of couple).

Find out your state's **penalty divisor ("B")** for one month. This can be obtained by calling your state's Department of Human Resources or whatever other division is responsible for determining financial eligibility for Medicaid in your state (see *State Medicaid Agency Contacts*, page 215).

Divide the **total amount of countable assets** by the total of the **net monthly expenses ("A")** plus the **penalty divisor ("B")**. This will give you the total number of months penalty you will be facing.

So far we have this:

Amount available ÷ (A + B) = # of months penalty.

Multiply the **number of months penalty ("C")** by the **penalty divisor ("B")**. This will give you the amount of the gift you can make: **C x B = gift amount.**

To see how the numbers work in two sample cases, see **Case Studies #1** and **#2**, beginning on page 167.

Why the Classic Half-A-Loaf Method No Longer Works

Unfortunately, the method described above will no longer work for gifts made on or after the date of enactment of the DRA, i.e., February 8, 2006. That is because if the person making the gift retains the "other half" of his or her assets, the penalty period will not even start to run until those assets are spent down. In other words, if Roland gives away $50,000 and retains $52,000, under the old rules the penalty period (10 months) starts to run on the date he makes the gift. He could then use the money he retained to pay privately for those 10 months, and then apply for Medicaid after the penalty period has expired, when he's down to his $2,000 exclusion amount.

But under the new rules, if Roland keeps $52,000 in the bank, the penalty period will not even start to run until he has spent down to $2,000, i.e., in 10 months. At that point, since he no longer has any assets (other than the $2,000 exclusion amount), he would have qualified for Medicaid *but for the gift penalty.* Roland, however, now has only $2,000, and is faced with a 10-month penalty. Clearly he cannot pay privately with the amount of money he has left. Thus, his family will wind up paying for him, using the $50,000 he gave them 10 months ago. At the end of the penalty period, his entire $100,000 will have been spent on his nursing home care, leaving his family with nothing. He's no better off than had he made no gifts at all.

New "Half-A-Loaf" Alternative Methods

There must be a better way! Well, there are several alternatives that take the new law into consideration. Let's take a look at them, now.

Gift + Return of Half the Assets

The simplest solution is for the Medicaid applicant to make the gift of all the excess assets, apply for Medicaid, and be turned down because of the gift. This starts the penalty period running. Then, the recipient(s) of the gift simply return "half" the assets back to the Medicaid applicant. This reduces the penalty period to half as long as initially imposed, and the applicant now has sufficient assets to pay privately for the penalty period. Note that the word "half" is in quotes: it rarely works out that the amount to transfer is exactly 50% of the amount of excess assets. You will need to follow the formula set out above to come up with the exact amounts to use.

The important consideration with this approach is that not all states permit the recipient of a gift to return less than the entire amount of the gift received as a way of reducing the penalty. If your state is an "all or nothing" state, then this technique is simply not available to you.

Gift + Annuity

By combining an outright gift to family members and a purchase of a Medicaid annuity with the balance of the countable assets, "half-a-loaf" planning can still be done. Here is how it works.

Example:

After Roland has calculated how much he should give to his children and how much he needs to retain in order to cover the resulting penalty period, he purchases a "Medicaid annuity" from an insurance company familiar with the Medicaid annuity rules. So if he had determined he needed to keep $50,000, then he purchases an annuity worth $50,000 and applies for Medicaid to start the penalty period. The annuity must pay back to him in equal payments over the penalty period, and each month he uses the annuity payment to cover his expenses.

NOTE: After making the above calculations, be careful that the annuity payments are not so high that the Medicaid applicant won't qualify for Medicaid, based on having too much income! See The "Too Much Income" Problem, immediately below.

Gift + Promissory Note

An alternative to the Gift + Annuity technique is the Gift + Promissory Note technique. The calculations are exactly the same, except that instead of having the Medicaid applicant use the excess funds to purchase an annuity, he or she loans those funds to a family member. In exchange for the loaned money, the family member signs a "Promissory Note" agreeing to pay back the loaned money over a specified time period (i.e., the number of months equal to the penalty period). According to the terms of the Note, each month a payment is made to the Medicaid applicant, who will then use that money to cover the nursing home expenses. As described in detail above (*Promissory Notes*, page 123), the loan must be documented in writing, all payments must be equal in amount, and the note must prohibit cancellation upon the lender's death.

NOTE: After making the above calculations, be careful that the Note payments are not so high that the Medicaid applicant won't qualify for Medicaid, based on having too much income! See the discussion below, *The "Too Much Income" Problem*.

The "Too Much Income" Problem

Whether utilizing an annuity purchase or a loan and Promissory Note combination, there is a possible trap to be aware of: since the payments of the annuity or Note each month are treated as "income" for Medicaid eligibility purposes, it is possible for the payments to be so high that the Medicaid applicant will have *too much income* to qualify for Medicaid. Not all states have this rule, but if they do, then it means that the penalty period will *not* start running at the time of the gift and will only start running after the payments from the annuity or Note are completed! That would be a disaster, because the Medicaid applicant will have no assets at that point, and yet be ineligible for Medicaid. Once again, the family members who received the gift money will have to turn around and use that money to pay the nursing home during the penalty period, leaving them nothing at the end.

To avoid this problem, the payments must be set so that they do not cause the Medicaid applicant's income—both his or her own income, such as from pension and Social Security *and* the annuity or Note income—to exceed the maximum income permitted by the state's rules. The family members who received the gift money will have to dip into those funds to cover the shortfall between the actual costs of the nursing home and the total permitted income of the Medicaid applicant. Coming up with the optimal amount of money to be gifted, while calculating the size of each payment, can be extremely complicated, with numerous interrelated moving parts, and will typically involve setting up a complex spreadsheet to work all this out. So do not be surprised by the legal bill to come up with the correct numbers: it is definitely not a trivial or easy task!

Gift of Interest in Home + Sale of Balance

As discussed above, an individual's home is an excluded asset (assuming the equity is under $500,000). However, upon the death of an individual who was covered by Medicaid, the state will want to be repaid for the Medicaid expenditures it made on behalf of that individual. The longer the owner has been in the nursing home, the greater the debt to the state. It's possible that it will take the entire value of the house to pay back the state.

How can the owner of the house, in this situation, preserve the greatest amount of value of the house, and still qualify for Medicaid in the shortest period of time?

One approach to protect at least part of the value of the home is as follows:

Owner of the home (who is in the nursing home) transfers 50% of the home to a child (or an irrevocable trust). Then owner applies for Medicaid. If owner has no other countable assets, owner will be eligible for Medicaid *but for the gift* of the interest in the home. Therefore, the penalty period will start running. Once the penalty is determined, the house can be sold. This will generate enough cash for owner to pay privately during the penalty period. Thus, 50% of the home's value has been protected. (Again, the actual percentage to be gifted away must be calculated by running through the "half-a-loaf" formula set forth above.)

Compare this to selling the home first, then making the gift and applying for Medicaid: in such case, since the Medicaid applicant will be sitting there with cash equal to half the proceeds of the house sale, applying for Medicaid will not start the penalty period running. That's because with all that cash, the applicant will not be Medicaid eligible *but for the gift* (the requirement to get the penalty period started). As a result, the applicant will have to go the additional step of using those proceeds to purchase an annuity (see page 105) or lending money to family members in exchange for a Promissory Note (page 123). Transferring the interest in the house first, then applying for Medicaid, and then selling the house, avoids those complications.

If the home has increased in value significantly since its purchase, the option of transferring the gifted portion of the house to a trust rather than outright to children will make more sense. In this case, the trust will be drafted as a so-called irrevocable "grantor trust." Such a trust reserves certain powers to the homeowner even after the interest is transferred to the trust, with the result that the homeowner is deemed the owner of the entire house for income tax purposes. The result of this technique is that upon the later sale of the house, the full $250,000 capital gains exclusion may be used. If the interest in the home had instead simply been gifted to one or more children, then the amount of taxes attributable to the gifted portion would *not* be eligible for this exclusion.

What if the homeowner still has some extra cash to spend down? A variation on the above is to transfer that cash *plus* a percentage interest in the home to children, apply for Medicaid, and then sell the home to obtain the cash to pay privately during the penalty period. Once again, the actual percentage to be gifted away must be calculated by running through the "half-a-loaf" formula set forth above, this time including both the cash and the value of the house in the gifted portion.

Exceptions:

The following transfers are exceptions to the general rule that penalizes transfers made by a person applying for Medicaid. Although these exceptions eliminate gift treatment for Medicaid purposes, they do not affect the possible *gift tax* cost of such a transfer (see page 56). For the transfers to trusts, it is recommended that the trust give a "limited power of appointment" to the grantor of the trust, which will eliminate any possible gift tax. (In addition, there is no gift tax that applies to outright gifts between spouses.)

Transfer to Spouse

A transfer between spouses is never penalized. After all, the assets of both spouses are added together when one spouse applies for Medicaid. Since it does not matter whose name the assets are titled in when the "snapshot" is taken, there is no reason to penalize a transfer of assets between spouses. Hence, it is a good idea to title all assets in the name of the Community Spouse as soon as it looks likely that the other spouse will be requiring nursing home care within a relatively short period of time.

Trust for the Sole Benefit of the Spouse

A transfer of assets by the Medicaid applicant to a trust for the "sole benefit" of the Community Spouse will not result in a penalty period. The spouse must be the sole beneficiary of the trust and payments must be made to or for the benefit of the spouse on a basis that is "actuarially sound" based on the spouse's life expectancy. One way to do that is to have distributions based on the same table that governs minimum distributions to a beneficiary of an IRA. Because a trust established by one spouse is deemed established by *either* spouse, such a trust is treated as if the Community Spouse set up the trust for him- or herself; under the trust rules discussed on page 59, the entire amount of the trust would still be countable as the Community

Spouse's own assets, should the Community Spouse ever need to apply for Medicaid also. Thus, the only reason for setting up such a trust is if the nursing home spouse wanted to limit the amounts that could be distributed to or for the benefit of the Community Spouse each year. Such limitations on distributions might be useful if the Community Spouse, for example, was not a good money manager or might easily be talked into foolish expenditures.

Transfer to Blind or Disabled Child

A transfer of assets to the Medicaid applicant's child who is legally blind or who is disabled as determined by Social Security rules (e.g., the child is receiving SSDI), will not result in a penalty period. However, if the child is disabled, be careful that the transferred assets do not cause the *child* to lose his or her government benefits as a result of the gift! The best way to make the gift yet protect the child's government benefits is to make the transfer into a trust for the child (see next paragraph).

Trust for the Sole Benefit of a Blind or Disabled Child

A transfer of assets by the Medicaid applicant to an irrevocable trust for the "sole benefit" of the applicant's blind or disabled child will not result in a penalty period. The child must be the sole beneficiary of the trust and payments must be made to or for the benefit of the child on a basis that is "actuarially sound" based on the child's life expectancy; one way to do that is to have distributions based on the same table that governs minimum distributions to a beneficiary of an IRA. Again, be careful that the transferred assets do not cause the *child* to lose his or her government benefits as a result of the gift! The trust must be set up as a "supplemental needs trust" by your attorney.

Upon the beneficiary's death, the balance of the trust will *not* have to be used to repay the state for any Medicaid outlays it made on behalf of the trust beneficiary. However, if the beneficiary dies before his or her normal life expectancy, leaving assets in the trust, those assets will be payable to the beneficiary's estate, where they will be subject to estate recovery (however, there is no estate recovery for benefits—other than nursing home care—that were provided to an individual under age 55).

Trust for the Sole Benefit of a Person Under Age 65

A transfer of assets by the Medicaid applicant to an irrevocable trust for the "sole benefit" of a disabled individual under age 65 will not result in a penalty period. This exception is not limited to trusts for children, so it could be for the use of a disabled grandchild, sibling, or other family member. The disabled individual must be the sole beneficiary of the trust and payments must be made to or for the benefit of the individual on a basis that is "actuarially sound" based on the individual's life expectancy. Once again, the trust must be worded carefully so that the transferred assets do not cause the disabled individual you are benefiting to lose his or her government benefits as a result of the gift.

Upon the beneficiary's death, the balance of the trust will *not* have to be used to repay the state for any Medicaid outlays it made on behalf of the trust beneficiary. However, if the beneficiary dies before his normal life expectancy, leaving assets in the trust, those assets will be payable to the beneficiary's estate, where they will be subject to estate recovery (however, there is no estate recovery for benefits—other than nursing home care—that were provided to an individual under age 55).

Transfer of the Home: Caretaker Child

A transfer of the home to the Medicaid applicant's child (of any age) will incur no penalty, if the child was living in the house *for at least two years* immediately prior to the date the parent was admitted to the nursing home, and the child provided care to the parent prior to the parent entering the nursing home that permitted the parent to delay entering the nursing home. The parent's home must be the child's sole residence during this period. The child will need to document (i) that the parent would have needed to move into a nursing home but for the child's assistance (a physician's assessment will be needed for this), and (ii) what the child actually did for the parent during this two-year period (keep good records!).

If the parent will need to be admitted into a nursing home before the child has cared for the parent for the full two years, then the parent will not be able to take advantage of the caretaker child exception. Also, if the child lives with the parent for over two years, but then moves out before the parent goes to a nursing home, this exception will not work: the two-or-more-year-period that the child takes care of the parent must immediately precede the parent's entry into the nursing home.

Although the federal statute does not explicitly deal with this, to be on the safe side, wait until the parent has entered the nursing home before making the transfer to the caretaker child. Until then, you won't know for certain whether you've met the two-year requirement.

Transfer of the Home: Resident Sibling

A transfer of the home to a sibling of the Medicaid applicant will incur no penalty, if the sibling has an equity interest in the home and was living in the house *for at least one year* immediately prior to the date the applicant was admitted to the nursing home. Note that care is not an issue, as it is with the "caretaker child" exception above.

Having an "equity interest" in the home means that the brother or sister must already own some percentage interest in the home at the time the balance of the home is gifted to him or her. The owner can deed a tiny percentage (1%) to the sibling who will be living there, but then should preferably wait at least one year before entering the nursing home in order to take advantage of this exception

It would be safer to wait until after the owner has entered the nursing home before making the transfer to the sibling. Until then, you won't know for certain whether the sibling has met the one-year requirement.

Transfer of the Home: Minor, Blind or Disabled Child

A transfer of the home to a child of the Medicaid applicant who is under age 21, blind, or disabled will incur no penalty (but see loss of benefit considerations, page 138).

Transfers Exclusively for Non-Medicaid Purposes

If you can prove that you made a gift purely for a purpose *other than* Medicaid planning, then even if the gift falls within the lookback period, it will be ignored.

You must present to the state convincing and objective evidence proving that the assets were transferred *exclusively* for a purpose other than to qualify or remain eligible for Medicaid. Transfers to avoid the Medicaid lien or estate recovery are included in the definition of Medicaid eligibility.

There is a rebuttable presumption that the transfers were made for purposes of Medicaid eligibility. In other words, if there was *any* expectation of applying for Medicaid that could reasonably be inferred to be a factor in your decision to transfer the asset, the presumption cannot be successfully rebutted. Merely stating that you were ignorant of the transfer penalty or verbal assurances that you were not considering Medicaid eligibility when the transfer was made are not sufficient. Nor can you rebut the presumption by stating that the transfers were done "for estate planning" or "for probate avoidance" purposes.

If the amount of your assets (and those of your spouse, if you are married) remaining after the transfer are sufficient to pay for medical (including long-term care) and living expenses reasonably expected to be incurred for you or your spouse for the next 60 months, then you should be able to claim that you certainly did *not* make the transfer for Medicaid planning purposes. After all, you had plenty of money to self-pay!

As to gifts you have not yet made, if you make gifts to, say, your grandchildren for their college education, or you buy a car for one of your children, or even make a large charitable donation, and at the time you're in good health and have sufficient assets to cover any possible long-term care for the next 5 years, you should document all of this at the time you make the gift. This information may come in handy should the unexpected happen and you or your spouse winds up applying for Medicaid within 5 years of the gift.

Hardship Waiver

Under the new Medicaid laws enacted in 2006, either the facility *or* the resident may petition the local Medicaid office for a hearing, to waive the imposition of the penalty from the earlier gifts made by the resident. The penalty period *may* be waived if:

- the individual is unable to obtain medical care without the receipt of Medicaid benefits,
- the gifted assets have been irretrievably lost and all reasonable avenues of legal recourse to regain possession of them have been exhausted, and
- application of the transfer penalty would deprive the individual of medical care such that the individual's health or life would be endangered or would deprive the individual of food, clothing, shelter or other necessities of life.

Assuming that relocating the nursing home resident back to his or her home would put the resident's life in jeopardy (since there may well be no one there to properly care for the resident), it should not be difficult to prove that the penalty from the prior gifts should be waived.

As you can see, the above procedures will put the resident and his or her entire family in a very precarious situation and cause much emotional turmoil for several months, while this whole thing is sorted out. Meanwhile, the family will have to incur significant legal fees to represent the resident in the hearing to waive the penalty. Accordingly, this is not something you would want to plan for!

Nursing Home Eviction Rules

If a nursing home resident has made gifts to family members, runs out of money after residing for some period of time in a nursing home, and a hardship waiver cannot be obtained, federal law permits the nursing home to evict the resident for non-payment, *if* the nursing home does all of the following:

- Prepares a summary of the resident's mental and physical health status;
- Prepares a post-discharge plan of care for the resident which will assist the resident to adjust to his or her new living environment; and

- Notifies the resident and a family member or legal representative of the resident of the pending discharge at least 30 days in advance of the discharge, letting them know of the resident's right to appeal the discharge action to the state.

The point of the above is that nursing home residents *can* be evicted from the facility for non-payment of their monthly fees. Accordingly, it is vital that the Medicaid rules be understood and followed, and appropriate appeals taken, in order to avoid this harsh result.

Transfers to Community Spouse

Since there is never a penalty for transfers between spouses, as a general rule a married couple should arrange to title as much of their assets as possible in the name of the Community Spouse, as soon as possible. Here are the reasons to do so:

- Once the CSRA is determined, any additional assets required to increase the Community Spouse up to that amount *must* be transferred from the nursing home spouse to the Community Spouse within one year of the Medicaid eligibility starting date.

- Should the nursing home spouse become incapacitated, it may be impossible to implement some of the techniques discussed in this book.

- For example, it may be possible to protect a substantial portion of the Community Spouse's assets even if the Community Spouse should die before the nursing home spouse. Such planning is not possible, however, if those assets are still in the incapacitated nursing home spouse's name at the death of the Community Spouse.

Purchase Long-Term Care Insurance, Make Gift

If you are able to qualify for long-term care insurance, consider purchasing a policy that has at most a five-year coverage option. Once the insurance is in place, make a gift of the maximum amount of assets you can afford to part with, considering your ongoing expenses and current income. If you need nursing home care within the five years, then you will have your bills covered by the policy and won't have to worry about the gift penalty. Once five years from the date of your gift has passed, you will be able to apply for Medicaid, since the prior gift is now outside of the lookback period. Thus, the most you'll ever have to pay the long-term care premiums is for five years. If possible, purchase a policy with decreasing coverage: in year 1 (the year you make the gift), you need coverage for five years; when you renew the policy in year 2, only for four years; in year 3, only for three years, etc. That way, you are not paying for more coverage than you need, because starting in year 6 you will be able to qualify for Medicaid, and you won't need the long-term care insurance coverage anymore.

If you already have long-term care insurance, be sure to take that into consideration when determining how much money you can give away. If you have coverage for five years, then you can make as large a gift as you wish to, since even if you have a stroke the next day and have to move into a nursing home, your long-term care insurance will cover you during the five-year lookback period. Upon the termination of the coverage of your insurance policy, you can apply for Medicaid, since the lookback period no longer includes the gifts you made more than five years ago.

What if you only have three-year coverage? Then you can still make a large gift, but you'll have to consider how you will pay privately for the two-year "gap" between the period covered by your insurance and the five-year lookback period.

/// **Example:**

Martha currently owns a long-term care policy that will pay for her nursing home care for up to three years. That means that if Martha has to move into a nursing home, the policy will pay her bills there for no more than three years. Since Martha's health is currently pretty good, she decides to make a large gift of her assets to her three children. However, she is careful to retain sufficient assets in her own name to cover the cost of the nursing home for the two-year period between when the insurance runs out and the lookback period no longer can count her gift. In other words, if Martha makes the gift and the next day has to go to the nursing home, her long-term care insurance policy will pay her bills there for the next three years. At the end of the three years she cannot apply for Medicaid, because that would cause a very long penalty period. Accordingly, she's set aside enough assets in her own name to cover the cost of a nursing home for a two-year period. This only matters if she enters the nursing home within the first two years, and with each passing month, that's one month fewer that she may have to pay for out of her own pocket.

Of course, it's possible that after two years Martha has not entered the nursing home. Since her three-year policy will now take her to the end of the lookback period, she does not have to worry about retaining assets to cover her care privately. So now she needs to dispose of the excess assets that she had set aside for the potential two-year gap. To avoid this problem, she could have given *all* her assets to her children, with the understanding (although not legally binding) that the children would pay for their mother's care if indeed she needed to enter the nursing home within the first two years.

Disclaiming an Inheritance

If a relative dies and leaves you (or your spouse) an inheritance, usually that's good news. But what if you're already on Medicaid? That money won't do you any good and will only disqualify you from the Medicaid program. You'd then have to spend down the inheritance till it's gone, and then reapply for Medicaid once you're broke. So much for the benefit of the inheritance!

Under state law, you can "disclaim" an inheritance or gift under a person's will, which means you refuse to accept the asset or money left to you. As a result, you're treated as if you never got the asset or money and it passes to the person next in line: if it was an inheritance (i.e., your relative died with no will), then it passes according to state law; if it was left to you under a will or trust, then it passes according to the terms of the will or trust. In most cases, it will pass to your children. In any event, the person making the disclaimer has no power over where the disclaimed money goes.

Unfortunately, the general rule is that for Medicaid purposes, the disclaimer is looked at as if you *did* receive the money and then turned around and gave it away. As a result, you'll be faced with a penalty for that gift.

Accordingly, the disclaimer won't accomplish what you hoped it would. In most cases, it's best if you accept the inheritance/gift, and then deal with it the same as any other countable asset, using one or more of the many techniques and options discussed in this book.

Chapter 15
POST-ELIGIBILITY ISSUES

Personal Needs Allowance

A nursing home resident on Medicaid is allowed to keep up to $60 or so per month, for personal expenses such as barber/beauty shop appointments, clothing, toiletries, and other miscellaneous personal expenses.

Health Care Expenses

Medical and remedial care expenses that are not subject to being repaid by an outside organization (such as a health insurance program) may also be deducted from the nursing home resident's income before paying the balance to the nursing home each month. Such expenses include Medicare and other health insurance premiums, deductibles, and coinsurance and necessary medical or remedial care recognized under state law but not otherwise covered under the state Medicaid program, subject to reasonable limits the state may establish on the amount of these expenses.

This is sometimes referred to as Post-Eligibility Treatment of Income (PETI). It would cover, for example, a hearing aid that was lost, and for which Medicare would not cover a replacement. The nursing home resident can put in a request with the state to have this expense covered out of the resident's own income. Assuming the request is approved, it would allow the resident to pay for the hearing aid instead of paying that money to the nursing home.

> In essence, Medicaid is paying for the hearing aid by permitting the resident to shift income from the nursing home to the hearing aid company.

Post-eligibility transfers by the Community Spouse

There is a split among the states on the treatment of transfers made by the Community Spouse *after* the nursing home spouse is determined to be eligible for Medicaid. Some states allow the Community Spouse to make such transfers without affecting the nursing home spouse's eligibility for Medicaid, but others treat it as if made by the nursing home spouse, thereby causing a period of disqualification. Often they make a distinction between a transfer of the house and that of other assets. Thus, you'll need to check with an experienced elder law attorney in your state to find out the current rule that applies to you, if you are thinking of doing such transfers. Of course, any such transfers will affect the Medicaid eligibility of the Community Spouse should he or she apply for Medicaid him- or herself after making such gifts, but that's a different question than if such gifts affect the eligibility of the *nursing home spouse*.

If the Community Spouse Dies First

If the Community Spouse dies before the nursing home spouse, the risk is that the assets owned by the Community Spouse will pass into the name of the nursing home spouse, causing the nursing home spouse to become immediately ineligible for Medicaid until the inherited assets are spent down. This often happens because the Community Spouse assumes he or she will outlive the nursing home spouse and never gives this any thought. Typically, the wills of the husband and wife leave everything to each other, if living, otherwise to the children. If they never had wills, then their state law would generally do the same thing, awarding all the assets to the surviving spouse. Accordingly, when the Community Spouse dies, all the assets that were protected as the CSRA are now handed over to the nursing home spouse, who of course has no use for them.

So what should the nursing home spouse do if the Community Spouse dies first, leaving all of his or her assets to the nursing home spouse? As discussed above (page 145), the nursing home spouse cannot simply "disclaim" (refuse) the inheritance or gift under the will. That will be treated as if the spouse received the assets and then made a penalty-causing gift of those assets. Instead, the best alternative in most cases is for the surviving spouse to accept the inheritance or gift under the will and then deal with the assets using one or more of the techniques discussed in this book.

However, to avoid this problem, the Community Spouse should create a new will, one that takes this problem into consideration.

Elective Share Problem

The first reaction of most people is to say, *"Well, why can't I just omit my spouse from my will entirely?"* While this can certainly be done, it will not be effective, because the laws of every state grant a surviving spouse certain minimum rights to the assets of the deceased spouse. The reason for this is to prevent a spouse from creating a will that leaves nothing to the surviving spouse, leaving that spouse impoverished and a ward of the state.

Each state has its own scheme to accomplish this by guaranteeing a surviving spouse some percentage of the deceased spouse's estate. This is called a spouse's "elective share" or "statutory share." The amount of the elective share depends on the laws of the state the couple resides in. Some states give a surviving spouse a one-third interest in the deceased spouse's estate no matter how long they were married. Other states use a gradually increasing percentage, e.g., 10% if married for under 2 years, 20% if between 2 and 4 years, 30% if between 4 and 6 years, etc., with a maximum of 50% if married 10 or more years.

If the Community Spouse tries to defeat the elective share by making gifts to children or other relatives, these gifts can be brought back into the calculation, depending on how long ago they were made and whether or not the other spouse consented to the gift. Some states apply the elective share to a so-called "augmented estate." This is an extremely complex set of rules that determines exactly which assets of the first spouse to die are subject to the elective share. In some cases, even assets that were given away years ago are brought back into this calculation, as are certain transfers to trusts. Just think of the last bald probate attorney you met—it's because he tore his hair out trying to figure out the elective share and augmented estate statutes!

Assuming that the Community Spouse will not have completely depleted his or her estate by death, a conservative approach, then, would be for the Community Spouse to write a new will, one that leaves *only the minimum amount necessary to satisfy the elective share* outright to the surviving (nursing home) spouse. The balance can safely be left to the children or other relatives. As you can see, this will give the spouse only half or a third (depending on the state law), immediately saving the other half or two-thirds of the assets from having to be spent down on nursing home care. This simple change can easily save thousands of dollars for the other family members!

The problem with the outright gift under the will is that not only does it cause the immediate disqualification of the surviving spouse from Medicaid benefits, but it exposes the full amount of the elective share to estate recovery, as assets of the surviving spouse. If the surviving spouse dies shortly after receiving the money, then most if not all of that money will wind up being paid over to the state under the estate recovery program, as reimbursement for its Medicaid payments (see *Estate Recovery*, page 155).

Thus, another approach is to leave the elective share amount in the form of a trust that satisfies the elective share statute yet will not be included in the surviving spouse's estate. The success of this approach depends not only on how the state permits the elective share to be structured, but also on how it handles estate recovery: some states limit recovery only to the probate estate, some go further. Again, this must be determined by an experienced elder law attorney in your state who can assist your travel through these very complicated waters!

The main point of the above is that it is not enough to qualify one spouse for Medicaid, without planning for the possibility that the Community Spouse may die first. Be sure that as part of your Medicaid planning your elder law attorney prepares a new will for the Community Spouse, one that deals with the "elective share problem" discussed in this section.

Change Beneficiary Designations

As discussed above, it is vital for the Community Spouse to change his or her will. But don't forget about investments that pass by beneficiary designation and *not* by will! This includes IRAs, 401(k)s, life insurance policies, and annuities. If any of these were retained as part of the Community Spouse's CSRA, be sure to change the beneficiary designation so it does not go directly to the nursing home spouse. Whether any of these need to fund the elective share trust discussed above or not is a difficult calculation that can only be determined by your elder law attorney, due to the variations in state law that affect the calculation of the elective share.

Divorce Option

One option that may be considered in order to protect the assets of the Community Spouse is a divorce. Often a couple is understandably reluctant to go this route, because of the social stigma of a divorce. However, if a spouse has Alzheimer's, advanced dementia, or other life-restricting illness, the undeniable fact may be that the couple's life together is already over, as a practical matter. A divorce at this point is not due to any lack of love between the two spouses but is purely for the financial protection of the Community Spouse; the nursing home spouse will be well-cared for via Medicaid payments. But without a divorce the Community Spouse's assets may be reduced to the point that the long-term welfare of the Community Spouse can be put in jeopardy.

That being said, some states may not allow a divorce from an incapacitated spouse. If they do, they probably will not permit all assets to be awarded to the Community Spouse. The general rule is that there must be an "equitable distribution" of the assets and income of the couple. The circumstances and needs of each spouse must be considered. If all the assets are awarded to the Community Spouse, the state Medicaid department could view that as a gift from the nursing home spouse, causing a period of ineligibility. However, if it is demonstrated that the nursing home spouse's bills will be well-covered by Medicaid, but the living expenses of the Community Spouse are not financed by government programs, there should be a good argument for awarding a greater percentage of the assets to the Community Spouse.

As you can see, you will need a good divorce attorney who must be guided by an experienced elder law attorney, to make this work! However, in the long run, it could positively affect the financial well-being of the Community Spouse without affecting the overall level of care of the nursing home spouse.

Post-Gift Transfers by Children

If you are going to make gifts to more than one child, it would be a good idea for the children to do one of the following after they receive the funds, assuming the plan is for the money to be kept available for your benefit should the need arise:

A. The children open up a joint bank account. Once the children receive the gift, they can make equal contributions of the funds you gave them into a joint bank account. It's important for them to document who contributed what, so that if one of the children is sued or divorced, only that child's share of the bank account can be attached by the creditor or divorcing spouse. In most cases, the account should be set up so that all contributing children must sign off on withdrawals, to protect against a child who falls on hard times (or temptation) and dips into the funds for personal use without telling the siblings. The advantage of this arrangement is that the money is segregated from the children's other assets, so they are more likely to use it for the parent's benefit, should the need arise. The disadvantage is, what if one of the children dies or become incapacitated? Who will succeed to the child's interest in the bank account? And will they go along with continuing to leave the deceased child's interest in that bank account? One partial solution would be to have each child sign a limited power of attorney to the other children, authorizing them to access the bank account if the first child becomes incapacitated.

B. The children create a joint trust. For even greater protection, once the children receive your gift, they can make equal contributions of the money you gave them into a single trust. One or more children can act as trustee although having an independent (i.e., non-family member) trustee will both better insulate the money from creditors of the children and hopefully avoid family squabbles on use of the funds. The trust can name you as beneficiary, to cover any of your "supplemental needs" (i.e., expenses *not* paid for by Medicaid, once you are eligible). This guarantees that the money will be available for you, should you ever need it, since it is now out of the children's names completely. Also, if a child is sued, divorced, or goes bankrupt, the share of your money you gave them is protected. Alternatively, the trust can allow distributions to be made *only* back to the children, who could then turn around and use it for your benefit, similar to the joint account arrangement discussed above. The advantage to this alternative is that it makes it much harder for the state to claim that the trust was "really" established by and for the parents, causing inclusion of the trust property in the parents' countable assets.

If the children are going to set up such a trust, it is important that they do *not* hire the same attorney who assisted you with your Medicaid planning. Also, the children should allow a reasonable amount of time to pass before they create and fund this trust. What's "reasonable"? Unfortunately, there is no hard and fast rule; clearly a week is too soon and five years longer than necessary, so somewhere in between! The attorney the children hire is in the best position to advise them about this issue. The reason for the above precautions is to make sure that the children's funding a trust for you is an independent act of theirs and not part of a coordinated plan that you and the children agreed to in advance of your gifts to them. Otherwise, the state Medicaid authorities can argue that in essence, *you* set up the trust *for yourself,* using your own money, and therefore all the assets in the trust are now countable under the self-funded trust rules!

Chapter 16
ESTATE RECOVERY

Upon the death of any individual who was covered by Medicaid while institutionalized (or a non-institutionalized Medicaid recipient who was at least age 55 at the time of receiving benefits), the state must seek to recover all of the expenditures it made on behalf of the now-deceased Medicaid recipient for nursing home costs, medical costs (hospital and prescription drugs) while in the nursing home, Medicare premiums and co-payments during this time, and HCBS payments.

Since this recovery is not made until after the death of the recipient, it is known as "estate recovery."

In essence, while you thought you had qualified for a government benefit, all you've really received is an interest-free loan! And upon your death, the government wants its loan paid back.

Prior to 1993, such estate recovery was optional—a state could implement it or not. However, in that year a new federal law was passed (known as OBRA '93) that mandated that every state *must* seek estate recovery from its Medicaid-receiving residents following their deaths. Interestingly, some states—such as Texas—managed to delay implementation of this federally mandated law until just recently, giving their citizens a break the rest of the states did not enjoy. And Michigan *still* has not implemented estate recovery!

Now if you're sharp, you may be thinking "Wait a minute…if someone qualifies for Medicaid, they have to be essentially broke. So where exactly is this money coming from to repay the state?" That's a good question, and the good news is that if your family member died owning nothing, then indeed the state is out of luck. It can't go after the kids' money. There must be some assets that the nursing home resident had a legal interest in, at the time of death, in order for the state to be repaid. That legal interest is defined as the "estate" of the deceased Medicaid recipient. However, how the word "estate" is defined varies from state to state, thereby affecting what assets the particular state can recover against.

Definition of "Estate"

All states must seek recovery at least from the "probate estate" of the Medicaid recipient. This is typically defined to include only assets that would pass by will. Such definition includes assets titled in the sole name of the decedent, but excludes assets that pass by beneficiary designation (such as a life insurance policy, annuity, IRA, 401(k), or similar plan payable to someone other than the insured's estate); POD (pay on death) bank accounts; TOD (transfer on death) stock certificates or brokerage accounts; trust property; joint bank accounts; and jointly owned real estate or other property that passes by operation of law automatically to the surviving owner(s) by right of survivorship.

Expanded Definition of "Estate"

Under the federal law, any state may adopt an expanded definition of "estate," to include any one or more of the following: assets conveyed to a survivor, heir or assign of the deceased individual through joint tenancy, tenancy in common, survivorship, life estate, living trust, or other arrangement (such as an annuity). In other words, the definition of "estate" could now include virtually any asset in which the deceased nursing home resident had any legal interest the moment before death. As of 2006, there are several states that have indeed passed laws adopting this expanded definition of "estate" for Medicaid estate recovery purposes. It is important that you know exactly what is and what is not subject to estate recovery in your particular state, so that you may plan accordingly.

Planning for Change

Unfortunately, even if you reside in a state that does not currently use an expanded definition of "estate," there is no guarantee that it may not do so at some time in the near future. Worse, a recent case held that there is no "grandfathering" for Medicaid recipients when the law changes midway through their nursing home stay: whatever law is in effect upon the death of a Medicaid recipient will apply, even if that means that assets which were not subject to recovery earlier in the recipient's nursing home stay are subject to recovery at the time of his or her death. This is another reason for only working with an elder law attorney who is not only active in his or her field and keeps up with legislation that may be introduced in your state affecting estate recovery, but who is also aware of trends in other states that may affect future legislation in your state. Of course, there is always the possibility that laws may change, and no attorney has a crystal ball, but you increase your odds of doing the best possible planning by working with a "plugged in" and savvy elder law attorney.

Exceptions

There are some exceptions that prevent estate recovery.

If you were under age 55 at the time you received Medicaid benefits *other than nursing home care*, then you will be exempt from estate recovery *for the amount of those benefits.*

No recovery may be made against your estate if you are survived by any of the following:

- your spouse
- a child of yours who is under age 21
- a dependent of yours who is blind or totally and permanently disabled, as defined under the Social Security regulations.

Note that unlike the TEFRA lien rules discussed below, it is not necessary that these individuals be living in your home for these exceptions to apply.

There will also be no recovery made against your home (i.e., it will *not* have to be sold to pay back the state) if:

1) a sibling of yours was living in the house for at least one year immediately prior to the date you were admitted to the nursing home and who has continuously lived in the house since then, or

2) if there is a son or daughter (of any age) of yours who was living in the house for at least two years immediately prior to the date you

were admitted to the nursing home, who has continuously lived in the house since then, and who provided care to you prior to your entering the nursing home which permitted you to delay entering the nursing home.

If all else fails, there's an exception to estate recovery if such recovery would work an "undue hardship" on the surviving family members. One example would be where the excluded asset is a working farm, and a forced sale of that farm would throw surviving family members out of work.

Timing of the Recovery Claim

Technically, the federal law states that recovery can be made "only after the death of the individual's surviving spouse." So if, for example, the surviving spouse dies a month after the Medicaid recipient spouse, a state *could* file a claim for recovery at that time. Many states, however, have taken a more liberal reading of this, and so long as there *is* a surviving spouse, no recovery will be made, no matter how long or short the surviving spouse lives. You'll need to check your own state's laws to find out which rule applies to your situation.

Notwithstanding the above, even in a state where recovery may be made after the surviving spouse's death, there typically is an additional limitation that applies to *all* claims against an estate: all states have a statute of limitations that bars claims against an estate that are made more than a certain number of months after the death. In many states, that limit is one year. So, in a state with such a law, if the surviving spouse dies more than a year after the Medicaid recipient spouse, it will be too late for the state Medicaid recovery unit to file its claim for estate recovery.

If a state can only file a claim when there is no child under 21, can it wait until the child attains age 21 and then file its recovery claim? Once again, this must happen within the statute of limitations period, assuming there's not a blanket exemption if there's a surviving child under age 21.

Procedure and Time Limit

If recovery is limited to the "probate estate," then the state must file a timely claim against the estate, just as any other creditor of the decedent must do. Many states limit this time period to file a claim to one year after the date of death. If the state files a claim for estate recovery too late, it is out of luck.

If a lien was filed against the house, however, the state may have a longer time in which to satisfy its claim (see *Liens*, page 164). Exactly *how* much longer depends on the lien law of your state; again, you would need to check with an elder law attorney in your state, but be prepared for the attorney not knowing the answer right off the bat, since this is an unsettled question in many states.

Sometimes the family of a deceased Medicaid recipient will attempt the "lay low" approach, not opening a probate estate and hoping that the limitations period will expire before the state files its claim. If that happens, then the family will indeed "win," since at that point it will be too late for the state to collect its money from the estate. However, many states have now implemented procedures where they are notified of the death of anyone in a nursing home who was a Medicaid recipient, and if probate of the estate is not opened by the family within 30 days, the state itself—as a creditor—will petition the court to open the estate, and then file its claim for estate recovery.

Waivers

In certain limited circumstances, the state must refrain from seeking recovery against the estate if it would result in undue hardship.

In addition, a state may waive recovery if it is not cost-effective. For example, the value of the house (or the amount to be recovered) may be small in relation to the administrative cost of seeking recovery.

Married Couples' Issues

In planning for estate recovery for a married couple, one must consider the possibility that either spouse may be the survivor.

If the Nursing Home Spouse Dies First

Following the death of the nursing home spouse, the state is limited to recovering assets in which the nursing home spouse had a legal interest. As a general rule, the state cannot go after assets that were owned by the surviving Community Spouse. A recent Illinois Supreme Court case backs this up.

A few states have begun to apply a "tracing" approach, whereby assets that once belonged to the nursing home spouse and were later transferred into the name of the Community Spouse can be reached by the estate recovery rules. This appears to be in violation of federal law.

If the Community Spouse Dies First

If the Community Spouse predeceases the nursing home spouse, the big issue is what happens to the assets owned by the Community Spouse upon his or her death. The last thing you want to have happen is for the assets to pass to the surviving spouse, who is in the nursing home on Medicaid. If that happens, the nursing home spouse will be immediately disqualified from receiving Medicaid, by virtue of being "over resourced," and any of those inherited assets still in the surviving spouse's name at his or her death will be subject to estate recovery. Accordingly, this possibility must be carefully planned for, because you never know which spouse may die first. (See detailed discussion beginning on page 149.)

Avoiding Estate Recovery

As discussed above, merely qualifying for Medicaid is not enough if upon your death your family will have to pay back the state every dime of benefits the state paid out on your behalf during your lifetime. However, there are some planning techniques you can implement.

CHAPTER 16

Eliminate Probate Assets

First of all, in states where estate recovery is only made by a claim against your probate estate (so-called "probate estate only" states), all you need be sure of is that the Medicaid recipient has *no* probate estate at death.

For example, you can title an automobile in joint names with a child. You don't even have to have a driver's license to be an owner of a car. So the car would be titled as "Mary Smith and John Smith, JTWROS." John is Mary's son, and upon Mary's death, sole title to the car passes automatically to him outside of probate. "JTWROS" stands for "joint tenants with right of survivorship." (Be sure to check your state's motor vehicle titling rules to be sure this will work in your state!) Since one car of any value is excluded during Mary's lifetime, it's protected during her life and escapes estate recovery on her death.

The same approach can even be taken for her house. Since a Medicaid recipient's house is normally excluded during her lifetime (up to $500,000 in equity value), it's only at the recipient's death that there's a problem. So to avoid the house being included in Mary's probate estate, she can title her house as JTRWOS with her son John, on her deed. CAUTION: Adding another person's name to the deed is a gift of an interest in the house, effective upon the date of the deed! Thus, when Mary has her attorney add her son John's name to the deed, she has just made a gift of 50% of the house to him. Although gift tax is rarely an issue, it should be considered. More importantly, though, is that this is a Medicaid-disqualifying transfer, with a large penalty attached. If Mary wants to go this route, she may be unable to apply for Medicaid for *five years* after she signs the deed.

Also, what if John is sued or divorced? Mary may still think of the entire house as "hers," but the creditor or divorcing spouse will view that 50% interest in the house as an asset of John's, and it could be subject to attack. Mary may find herself out on the street if the house has to be sold to satisfy the judgment or divorce settlement.

Some states permit adding another person to a deed while giving them less than 50%. Ideally, you would want to give your child as small a percentage interest in the house as possible, yet still have the house pass to the child upon your death via the right of survivorship. For example, a 1% joint interest would reduce the amount of the gift as well as expose less of your house to the child's creditors. However, sometimes the rule for real estate law purposes differs from the rule for Medicaid purposes. So, a word to the wise: be sure that the attorney who is doing the new deed for you is up-to-date on the effect that will have on your Medicaid eligibility! (See page 95 for more on this topic.)

Transfer House Shortly Before Death

If the Medicaid recipient—or other family member if the recipient is incapacitated—transfers the home shortly before death, the home will no longer be part of the deceased Medicaid recipient's estate, and thus will escape recovery.

Such a transfer will cause the imposition of a period of ineligibility, requiring the family to pay privately for the nursing home care during this period. However, this may be a small price to pay to avoid the much larger bill of estate recovery.

Example:

Mildred, a widow, is nearing the end of her life. She has been in the nursing home for five years. If she died today, the state would seek reimbursement from her estate of approximately $285,000, for which it would look to her house. Instead, her family deeds the house to themselves using a durable power of attorney that specifically authorizes such gifting, and the family dutifully reports the gift to the state. Because of this gift, she is immediately disqualified from Medicaid and her family must now pay for her final months in the nursing home. Upon Mildred's death, she no longer owns the home, leaving nothing for the state to attach in satisfaction of its estate recovery claim. Of course, if the state had already filed a lien against the house (see below), then this technique would not work.

Some states may claim that such a transfer of the home is a **"fraudulent transfer."** A "fraudulent transfer" is a transfer of property by a person for the purpose of defeating, hindering, or delaying the person's creditors. If a state were successful in making such a claim, all it would mean is that the house would have to be retransferred to the Medicaid applicant and once again would be subject to estate recovery. The family would be no worse off than it would have been had it done nothing. Unlike actual "fraud" against the state (such as hiding assets and not reporting them to the state on a Medicaid application), which can result in criminal or civil penalties, a "fraudulent transfer" carries no such penalties. It is also possible that the fraudulent transfer rules do not apply to transfers in a Medicaid context, since there are already specific federal statutes within the Medicaid sections that set forth the penalties for gifts, which would trump the fraudulent transfer rules. Needless to say, you should consult with an attorney before doing anything like this.

Liens

To prevent Medicaid recipients from disposing of their assets prior to death, thereby avoiding the state's attempt at estate recovery, states are permitted to file "liens" against certain property of a Medicaid recipient.

> A lien (pronounced "lean") against your home is a recorded document filed by a creditor of yours that prohibits the sale of your home without first satisfying the existing debt. It is similar to a mortgage, which prohibits you from selling your house without first paying off the bank. In the Medicaid context, it is filed by the state to guarantee repayment of all the money it will pay out for your care while you are on the Medicaid program.

Under the Tax Equity and Fiscal Responsibility Act of 1982 (known as "TEFRA"), states have the option of imposing liens to ensure repayment of their Medicaid expenditures. Thus, the state you live in may or may not impose liens.

When Applied

Following notice and opportunity for a hearing, a lien may be placed on the home of the Medicaid recipient once it is established that the recipient is not expected to return to his or her home. Note that this should not be confused with the continued exclusion of the home, no matter how likely it is as a practical matter that the Medicaid recipient will ever return home, so long as the "intent to return home" is maintained. In other words, the state can determine that you are both *unlikely* ever to return to your home for TEFRA lien purposes and *likely* to return home for Medicaid eligibility purposes!

The lien may be filed no matter how old you are, so long as you are receiving Medicaid for nursing home or home and community based services (HCBS). Recovery may only be made after the death of the Medicaid recipient or, if sooner, upon the sale of the home.

Exceptions

The lien may not be *imposed* at the time any of the following are lawfully residing in your home:

- your spouse
- a child of yours who is under age 21
- a child of yours who is permanently blind or disabled, as defined under the Social Security regulations
- a brother or sister of yours who has an equity interest in your house and who has lived there at least one year prior to your entering the nursing home.

The lien may not be *enforced* if any of the following are lawfully residing in your home and *have been* lawfully residing in your home since the date you entered the nursing home:

- a child of yours who lived there at least two years prior to your entering the nursing home and whose care allowed you to delay your going there; or
- a brother or sister of yours (who may or may not have an equity interest in your house) who has lived there at least one year prior to your entering the nursing home.

Finally, the lien must be removed if you leave the nursing home and actually move back home.

Chapter 17

CASE STUDIES

THE FOLLOWING ARE "CASE STUDIES," OR EXAMPLES OF THE THINKING THAT A SHARP ELDER LAW ATTORNEY WOULD GO THROUGH IN ANALYZING THE ISSUES OF ACTUAL CLIENTS AND COMING UP WITH REALISTIC SOLUTIONS. GOING THROUGH THEM WILL HELP YOU SYNTHESIZE AND LEARN HOW TO APPLY MANY OF THE VARIOUS TECHNIQUES DISCUSSED IN THIS BOOK.

Study #1:

Single Person with $215,000 in assets, no home, and $2,090 monthly income.

George is single and has the following assets:

CDs	$100,000
Bank accounts	5,000
IRAs	110,000
2001 auto (Kelly Blue Book value)	12,000

Here is his monthly income:

Social Security	$990
Federal retirement pension	1,100
CD interest	250

His monthly expenses:

Nursing home fee	$5,500
Health insurance premiums	200
Miscellaneous (haircuts, toiletries, magazines, etc.)	100

Let's go through this step-by-step.

- **Total Assets.** The auto is excluded, so we don't count it for this purpose. That leaves a total of $215,000 of countable assets. He is allowed a personal exclusion of $2,000, so the amount he must "spend down" is $213,000.

- **Net Monthly Expenses.** The total of his typical monthly expenses is $5,800. From this we subtract his income. We don't count his investment income of $250 for this purpose, since the assets that generate this income will be depleted soon, so his countable income is $2,090 per month. Thus, his monthly out-of-pocket expenses come to $5,800 - $2,090 = $3,710. In other words, he has to dip into his savings each month to cover this shortfall of $3,710.

- **First Thoughts.** Since George is already in the nursing home, his planning options are somewhat limited. He cannot make gifts and wait five years until the expiration of the lookback period; that would be too expensive. However, he can always reduce his countable assets by making gifts to family members using the "half a loaf" technique discussed on page 130, because that would allow him to qualify for Medicaid much sooner. So let's take a look at how to calculate that.

- **Penalty Divisor.** After checking with his state Medicaid office, he finds out that his state's penalty divisor is $5,000.

- **Calculating the Proper Size of Gift.** Dividing the total amount of George's countable assets ($213,000) by the total of his net monthly expenses ($3,710) + the penalty divisor ($5,000) gives us this:

$213,000 ÷ (3,710 + 5,000) = $213,000 ÷ 8,710 = 24.45,
or approximately 24.5 months' penalty

Multiply the above number of months' penalty (24.5) x the penalty divisor ($5,000) = $122,500. Thus, **he should make a gift of $122,500 and use the balance of his assets ($90,500) to purchase a Medicaid-friendly annuity.**

George must immediately apply for Medicaid. Since he still possesses $90,500 too much, he will be denied, but this step is necessary in order to get the penalty period started.

The annuity will pay George $3,710 per month for the 24.5 month period. The annuity, combined with his Social Security and pension income, will be sufficient to cover his nursing home bill during the penalty period. Upon the expiration of the 24.5-month penalty period, the annuity payments stop, and George can now re-apply for Medicaid. Because all of his assets will be gone by then, he will qualify for Medicaid at that time.

NOTE ON INCOME CAP RULES: In some states, George's total income ($5,800) will be too high for him to qualify for Medicaid without him funneling his income through a "Miller Trust" (see discussion beginning on page 24). Even then it may *still* be too high for him to qualify for Medicaid. And it is important for George to be able to qualify for Medicaid *but for the penalty-causing gift*, in order to start the penalty period running. In such case, the amount of the annuity will have to be adjusted so that the monthly payments to George cause his total income to be just under the "income cap" amount. Since that will not give him enough money each month to cover his nursing home cost, his family will have to dip into the money he already gave them to cover this shortfall during the penalty period. As you can see, these calculations have a lot of moving parts, and they *must* be made by an experienced elder law attorney if this approach is to be successful.

⁄⁄⁄ Proof:

If George decides to make this gift of $122,500, he will have $90,500 left in his name. His cost of living for the 24.5-month penalty period (above what he can cover with his income) will be $3,710 per month x 24.5 = $90,895. That leaves him with an excess of $395. Undoubtedly the nursing home costs will increase over the two-year period when he will be paying privately, so it's doubtful he will have too much money at the end of the period.

⁄⁄⁄ Result:

By making this gift, George has protected over $122,000 for his family, while qualifying for Medicaid sooner.

NOTE: His Social Security and pension income will continue to be paid to the nursing home even after he is on Medicaid. The Medicaid program will simply pick up the difference between these income payments and the actual nursing home costs.

What If George Is Not Yet In The Nursing Home?

As you can see from the above example, once George is in the nursing home, any gift has a penalty period that results in George having to pay out of his own pocket until the penalty period expires. Even though George saved over $122,000, he still had to spend over $90,000 of his money before he qualified for Medicaid. If he had made the gift earlier, he could have protected it *all* for his family.

So let's assume that George is not yet in the nursing home, but wants to plan ahead. Assume his assets and income are the same. The only difference will be his monthly living expenses. Since he's living at home, he won't have the nursing home bills, but he will certainly have grocery and restaurant expenses, he may be driving his car, he may even need to hire part-time assistance as his health worsens. Unfortunately, this calculation forces George to guess how many months he will remain at home, not needing to move to the nursing home. If he makes a larger gift and needs to go to the nursing home sooner than anticipated, then his family will have to use some of the gifted assets for his care. If he remains in better health than he thought, then he may have money left over at the end of the penalty period. Such calculations are at best an educated guess, based on George's expected health and financial needs. However, it is almost always better to come close than to do nothing! Once again, the assistance of an experienced elder law attorney is absolutely necessary to thread the family through all of these options.

- **Auto.** As discussed above (see *Estate Recovery*, page 155), merely qualifying for Medicaid is not the end of the story, if there are any excluded assets owned by the Medicaid recipient at the time of his or her death. In George's case, planning must also be done to protect George's auto against estate recovery, keeping in mind the extent of the state's ability to reach George's "estate" following his death.

George can simply retitle his auto into joint names with one of his children (page 162). Also, if he will not need the auto anymore, he can give it to one of his children. In either case, he is making a gift. However, since the auto was an excluded asset, there is no penalty: there is never a penalty for gifting an excluded asset (other than the home).

Study #2:

Single person with $42,000 in assets, a home, and $900 monthly income.

Maria is single and has the following assets:

Bank accounts/CDs	$42,000
Home	250,000
2001 auto (Kelly Blue Book value)	12,000

Here is her monthly income:

Social Security	$900

Her monthly expenses:

Nursing home fee	$5,500
Health insurance premiums	200
Miscellaneous (haircuts, toiletries, magazines, etc.)	100

Let's go through this step-by-step.

- **Total Assets.** The home and auto are excluded, so we don't count them for this purpose. That leaves a total of $42,000 of countable assets. She's allowed to keep up to $2,000 as her personal exclusion, so really her "spenddown" amount is actually $40,000.

- **Net Monthly Expenses.** Adding up her typical monthly expenses, the total is $5,800. From this we subtract her income. Thus, her monthly out-of-pocket expenses come to $5,800 - $900 = $4,900. Clearly, she cannot afford the nursing home without outside help, be it from Medicaid or family.

- **Medicaid Eligibility.** Without doing any planning, Maria's remaining savings will be completely gone in a little over 8 months. At that point, she should immediately qualify for Medicaid coverage of her nursing home bills. Maria's Social Security income will continue to be paid to the nursing home even after she is on Medicaid. The Medicaid program will simply pick up the difference between her income and the nursing home cost.

- **First Thoughts.** Although Maria does not have a lot of savings, there is no reason to just spend it until it's gone. With relatively small amounts of countable cash, setting up a half-a-loaf strategy may not be cost-effective, because of the complexity and legal fees involved. Instead, she should try to spend down her extra $40,000 by the following:
  - improve her house (page 75)
  - upgrade her auto (page 77)
  - pre-pay her own funeral and burial expenses (page 39)
  - pre-pay burial spaces for other family members (page 40)

If there is still any money left after the above, she can certainly utilize the "half-a-loaf" method to gift half of that balance and use a promissory note or Medicaid annuity for the other half. Alternatively, Maria can retain the balance of her savings to pay privately for a few months, and then apply for Medicaid coverage. Sometimes that will help her move up closer to the top of the waiting list for the nursing home and secure placement sooner.

- **Estate Recovery.** As far as Maria is concerned, getting herself placed in an excellent nursing home should be her top priority. She cannot afford to reside in a facility that does not accept Medicaid payments unless she is willing to sell her house to cover those costs (which could easily exceed the entire value of her house in a few years). Fortunately, there are many excellent facilities that accept both private pay and Medicaid. So if Maria does Medicaid planning or not, her situation really will not be that much different.

On the other hand, her family will lose not just $40,000 if Maria does no planning, but thousands more due to estate recovery upon her death. Thus, if she lives for another 5 years, her estate will owe the government 60 months x $4,900 = $294,000. Unless her house has appreciated in value beyond that amount, the state will require her house to be sold and the entire proceeds paid over to them, leaving her family with nothing. As you can see, Maria's family really has more at stake than she does, so avoiding estate recovery should become the main focus of any Medicaid plan for Maria.

Since the only asset Maria will possess at her death is her home, let's take a look at some of the options of avoiding estate recovery against her home.

Possible Solutions

1) **Gift house five years in advance.** At least five years before Maria thinks she may need nursing home care, she deeds the house to her children. She can continue to live in the house, with the permission of her children. Since the lookback period is five years, so long as she does not apply for Medicaid before that date the gift will be ignored. Upon her death, since she no longer owns the house, it is protected against estate recovery.

This could be risky, though: what if one of the children gets sued or divorced? A child's interest in the house can then be reached by these creditors, possibly forcing a sale. If Maria no longer has legal ownership, she could wind up on the street.

2) **Gift joint interest in house.** Maria can add one or more children onto her deed, ensuring that each owner is a "joint tenant with right of survivorship" or "JTWROS." That form of ownership ensures that upon Maria's death, her interest evaporates and avoids estate recovery (unless she lives in a state with an "expanded estate recovery" statute). She still must wait out the five-year lookback period, though. Another disadvantage is that she is a co-owner of the house with the children, so she cannot sell it without their permission and if they are sued or divorced, the child's interest in the house could be attached, once again possibly causing her to lose her ability to live in her home.

In some states, it is possible to have unequal joint tenancy interests. If such is the case, then a tiny percentage interest can be given away, such as 1%, causing a very small gift (see page 96). Then, when Maria applies for Medicaid, she will only be faced with less than a month's penalty. Her children would certainly be willing to pay that cost, in exchange for her protecting the entire value of the house by virtue of the joint ownership deed.

3) **Transfer house to trust.** Maria can also transfer the house into an irrevocable trust. The advantage is that she can continue to control the house, by serving as sole trustee, yet protect it against creditors of her children. There can be no estate recovery against the trust, since Maria gave up ownership in the house on the date she deeded it into the trust. She can retain a right to live in the house for her lifetime, by putting that requirement right into the trust document. That can actually be useful for income tax purposes, since it will cause the basis of the house to be re-adjusted to the value as of Maria's death; that can save the children capital gains taxes when they go to sell the house after Maria's death. Once again, though, Maria will have to wait out the five-year lookback period before applying for Medicaid.

4) **Gift house, retain life estate.** To protect Maria's right to continue to live in her house as long as she is able, and to protect it against creditors of her children, she can deed just a "remainder interest" in the house to her children (or to an irrevocable trust). Another way to think of this type of deed is that she is giving the house to her children (or the trust) but retaining a "life estate" in the house; that's what protects her lifetime interest to live in the house. She still must wait out the five-year lookback period, though. On her death, there can be no estate recovery against the house (unless she lives in a state with an "expanded estate recovery" statute that includes life estates).

5) **Sell house, move in with child.** If Maria thinks that she may need to move into a nursing home before five years but after at least one year, Maria can sell her home and purchase an interest in the home of one of her children. She can structure this either as a purchase of a life estate in the child's home or a purchase of a joint interest.

- **PURCHASE OF LIFE ESTATE.** Maria can purchase a life estate in the child's home. By looking up her age in the life estate table (page 207), she can calculate the percentage of the child's home she needs to buy for her $250,000 to avoid making a gift to the child. So if Maria is age 80, her life estate is worth 0.43659 (43.659%) according to the table. If she has $250,000 to invest in the child's house, then she can purchase a life estate in a house worth $572,620 ($250,000 ÷ 0.43659).

Of course, the chances of her child's house being worth exactly that amount are extremely unlikely. If the child's house is worth less than that, Maria will be making a gift to the child who owns the house if she gives the child $250,000. That is because at age 80, her life estate is worth 43.659% of the value of whatever house she owns a life estate in. So if the $250,000 is worth more than 43.659% of the value of the entire house, she's paying more for her life estate than she needs to. For example, if the child's house is only worth $400,000, she only needs to pay the child 43.659% of $400,000, or $174,636, for a life estate in the entire home. If she pays $250,000 for that life estate, she's essentially overpaying by $75,364; that amount is a gift to the child. If she did that, she'd have to wait five years to avoid a penalty on the amount of that gift. On the other hand, if the house is worth more than $572,620, then she will be buying a life estate in less than 100% of the house; in that case, it's easy for the deed to adjust for that.

In any case, upon her death, her interest terminates, leaving the home once again titled 100% in the name of the child (or child and child's spouse, if that's how the house was formerly titled).

NOTE: If Maria does not live in the house for at least one year after she signs the deed, then her purchase of the life estate will be deemed to be a gift to her child of the entire $250,000, for Medicaid purposes (see page 101). Thus, this should only be done if she feels fairly certain, based on her current health, that she will not need nursing home care for at least one year.

- **PURCHASE OF JOINT INTEREST.** To avoid the requirement that Maria live in her child's home for at least one year in order to avoid having the purchase treated as a gift, she can instead purchase a joint interest in the child's home. If the child's home is valued at, say, $500,000, Maria can purchase a 50% joint interest (with a right of survivorship) in the child's home and move in. Since Maria is paying her child the fair market value of a 50% interest in the home, it's not a gift, so there's no penalty period to worry about. After a reasonable period of time, should Maria need to go to a nursing home, her interest in her child's home will be an excluded asset. Although there is no "one year requirement" for the joint purchase, clearly the longer she is there, the better. Upon her death, the interest passes to the child under the deed, by operation of law, and there is no estate recovery against the house (unless Maria lives in a state that has an expanded definition of "estate" that includes joint property).

6) **Effect of lien.** If Maria lives in a state that allows for the filing of a lien against the house of a Medicaid recipient, the general rule going back hundreds of years (the so-called "common law" of the United States) is that the lien on a person's joint property interest is extinguished when that person dies and the right of survivorship passes to the other joint owner(s). Thus, ordinarily, the state is out of luck trying to enforce its lien to collect estate recovery against the property that is now owned 100% by the surviving joint owner(s). However, to be on the safe side, Maria should check with an attorney in her state to see if a specific statute was passed that overrules the common law rule just stated. Certainly if Maria has given the house away (either outright to her children or to an irrevocable trust) and does not own the house at her death, no lien can attach to it. But if she does any of the other options discussed above, there is the possibility that the lien may take precedence over any joint owner's interest, at her death.

7) **Crisis planning.** If Maria is already in the nursing home and has done no planning with the house, is she out of luck?

If she lives in a state where a small percentage joint tenancy gift can be made, that's probably her best bet (see page 96).

Otherwise, she will probably have to sell the house and do some of the other techniques discussed in this book, such as half-a-loaf gifting, etc. She should definitely consider the *Gift to Trust of Interest in Home + Sale of Balance* technique discussed on page 135.

If she does nothing, many states have a law that permits a "lien" to be placed on the house after six months. (See page 164.) The lien prevents the house from being sold unless the state is first reimbursed for its Medicaid payments on Maria's behalf. If that happens, then the family will have to face up to repaying the state for Maria's Medicaid coverage, after her death. The family will either keep her home and pay off the state (whereupon it will file a Release of Lien) or sell the home and pay back the state. In any event, if Maria's estate recovery bill *exceeds* the value of the house, the family is *not liable* for the shortfall.

Study #3:

Married Couple with $200,000 in assets, a home, and $2,500 monthly income: CRISIS PLANNING!

Mark and Isabelle are married. Isabelle recently moved into a nursing home, and Mark continues to live in the family home.

Here are their combined assets:

Bank accounts and CDs	$10,000	W*
IRA	50,000	H
Variable annuity	50,000	H
Mutual funds	90,000	JT
Home	250,000	JT
2001 auto (Kelly Blue Book value)	12,000	W

*Owned by husband (H), wife (W), or jointly (JT)

Their monthly income:

Social Security	$900	W
Social Security	1,200	H
Pension	400	H

Their monthly expenses:

Nursing home fee for Isabelle	$5,500
Health insurance premiums	200
Miscellaneous (haircuts, toiletries, magazines, etc)	100
Upkeep of house (average)	600
Food for Mark	350

Let's go through this step-by-step.

- **Total Assets.** The home and auto are excluded, so we don't count them for this purpose. Everything else is added up, regardless of whose name it is titled in: husband's, wife's or joint. Thus they have $200,000 in countable assets.

- **Net Monthly Expenses.** The couple's typical monthly expenses total $6,750. From this we subtract their combined income of $2,500. As you can see, they are short $4,250 each month. At this rate, this couple will be completely broke in less than four years if they do nothing. A better idea is to do some Medicaid planning!

- **Medicaid Eligibility**

  - **ASSETS.** Upon Isabelle's entry to the nursing home, Mark should request a Spousal Assessment (i.e., a "snapshot") from the Medicaid department of his state, in which it determines exactly how much he can keep (his "CSRA"). Since the combined assets of both spouses exceed the current CSRA of $101,640, that is the amount he will be allowed to keep (assuming he's in a "100% state"); the balance of their assets, other than Isabelle's $2,000 personal exclusion, will have to be spent down or otherwise depleted before Medicaid will pay Isabelle's nursing home bills. Thus, they have $96,360 "too much" money to qualify for Medicaid ($200,000 – $101,640 – $2,000).

  - **INCOME.** Once Isabelle is eligible for Medicaid, Mark is entitled to have income of *at least* $1,650 per month. Since his Social Security and pension total only $1,600 per month, he will be allowed to keep $50 of his wife's income each month; the rest of Isabelle's income will have to be paid to the nursing home (less a small monthly "personal needs allowance" of $50-70 and occasional payments for certain medical expenses not covered by Medicaid). The Medicaid program will pick up the difference between her income and the nursing home cost.

- **Estate Recovery.** Getting Isabelle on Medicaid is not the end of the problem. Even if Isabelle qualifies, the state will want to be repaid every dollar it spent on her care, following her death. Thus, some consideration must be paid to avoiding this "estate recovery." Otherwise, if Mark predeceases Isabelle and the house passes into her name alone, the house may have to be sold to repay the state, leaving her children little or nothing.

■ **What to Do First.** Because Isabelle's mental condition may deteriorate to the point where she can no longer legally sign anything, it is a good idea immediately to take her name off all assets, so that Mark is the sole owner. This does not change the CSRA calculation, but it will permit Mark to make purchases and gifts even after Isabelle becomes incapacitated.

■ **How to "Spend Down" the $96,360 "Excess Assets".**
  ■ Prepay funeral and burial expenses of both spouses (page 39): estimated cost: $12,000
  ■ Prepay burial expenses of other family members (page 40): estimated cost: $3,000
  ■ Improve the house (page 75): estimated cost: $15,000 (new heater/AC, new roof, etc.)
  ■ Buy a newer auto for Mark (page 77): estimated cost: $10,000 plus trade-in of old car
  ■ Buy additional personal property (big screen TV, computer, grand piano, etc.) (page 38): estimated cost: $6,000
  ■ Make a gift using the half-a-loaf technique (page 130); see below for calculations

■ **Half-A-Loaf Gifting.** After making the above expenditures of $46,000, there is still $50,360 of excess assets, before Isabelle will qualify for Medicaid. By making a gift of $27,500 to the children and using the $22,860 balance of the "excess" to purchase an annuity or lend to the children in exchange for a promissory note, there will be a penalty period of 5.5 months (assuming the state "divisor" is $5,000).

■ **Here's the Formula for the Amount of the Gift:** Divide the total amount of excess assets ($50,360) by the total of the couple's net monthly expenses ($4,250) + the penalty divisor ($5,000), which gives us this:

$$\$50,360 \div (4,250 + 5,000) = \$50,360 \div 9,250 = 5.44,$$

or approximately 5.5 months' penalty (most states will round up).

Multiply the above number of months' penalty (5.5) x the penalty divisor ($5,000) = $27,500. Thus, **Mark should make a gift of $27,500 to the children and use the balance of their excess assets ($22,860) to purchase a Medicaid-friendly annuity or lend to the children in exchange for a promissory note.**

Mark should then immediately apply for Medicaid for Isabelle, whereupon he will be told that because of the gift, Isabelle is disqualified for 5.5 months (of course, he already expected that, but he had to apply in order to get the penalty period running).

The annuity/note payments will increase Mark's monthly income for that 5.5-month period, allowing him to cover the private cost of Isabelle's nursing home residency, and at the end of the period, he will have just below the CSRA of $101,640.

Proof: 5.5 months x $4,250 = $23,375. Since this is slightly more than the retained amount of $22,860, he will be slightly short in the final month. Typically, the children will pay this small amount out of the $27,500 gift they received at the beginning of this process.

At that point, he can re-apply for Medicaid on behalf of his wife, and, the penalty period having expired, she will immediately qualify, and all her nursing home bills will be paid by Medicaid.

Thus, *these techniques will save the family $72,985 out of the original excess of $96,360.* Not bad for a "crisis" situation, where no advance planning had been done! Compare that to not doing anything and simply spending down the "excess assets" on Isabelle's nursing home care, which would have left the family with $-0-!

■ **Estate Recovery Issues**

As mentioned above, qualifying Isabelle for Medicaid is only half the battle. We must also plan for eventual estate recovery upon her death.

If she is the first to die, then there can be no estate recovery while Mark is still living, since federal law prevents a state from attempting to recover against the assets of a surviving spouse. However, upon

Mark's later death, some states may attempt to seek reimbursement from a portion of his estate, under the theory that part of his estate really belonged to Isabelle; this depends on how they define "estate" within their state statutes and regulations.

In this case, the big asset is their house. Let's take a look at some of their options.

■ **How to Protect the House.** Let's first look to see what would happen if Mark and Isabelle did nothing with the house.

   ■ **Isabelle Dies First.** If Isabelle dies first and the home is still titled in joint names, some states will be able to file a recovery claim against her 50% interest. Most states, however, only look to the probate estate of the Medicaid recipient, so in those states, no recovery would be possible. If Isabelle dies first and the home has already been titled in Mark's name, then most states would not be able to make a claim against Isabelle's former interest in the home. In any event, no claim may be filed while Mark is still living.

   ■ **Mark Dies First.** If Mark is the first to die and the home is still titled in joint names, the house will pass into Isabelle's sole name. Thus, it will be part of her probate estate and subject to estate recovery in all states after she dies. That can cause a loss of the entire value of the home, depending on how long Isabelle lives while on Medicaid. If instead the home is retitled into Mark's name alone, then he may be able to leave Isabelle only a percentage interest in the house (and any other assets still in his name), enough to satisfy the "elective share" either outright or in a trust under his will (see page 150).

   ■ **Gift Joint Interest in House.** Once the house is in Mark's name alone, he may be able to add one or more children onto the deed, ensuring that each owner is a "joint tenant with right of survivorship." That form of ownership ensures that upon Mark's death, his interest will not form part of the elective share amount. (NOTE: Elective share calculations can get very complex, since each state figures the elective share differently and may have laws that ignore gifts by one spouse that reduce the elective share owed to the other spouse. This is definitely something your elder law attorney must figure out for you!) Assuming Isabelle is already on Medicaid, it is probably okay for Mark to make a gift of an interest in the house to their children without affecting Isabelle's eligibility. As discussed above, Mark needs to be aware that once he adds children to the deed, they are co-owners of the house with him, so he cannot sell it without their permission and if they are sued or divorced, the child's interest in the house could be attached, possibly causing him to lose his ability to live in the home.

In some states, it is possible to have unequal joint tenancy interests. If such is the case, then a tiny percentage interest can be given away, such as 1%, causing a very small gift. This can be important if a gift by Mark does indeed affect the eligibility of Isabelle. In that case, it would be important to make the gift as small as possible. Then, when Isabelle applies for Medicaid, she will only be faced with a very small penalty. The family would certainly be willing to bear that cost, in exchange for protecting the entire value of the house by virtue of the joint ownership deed. (See page 96.)

- **Gift House, Retain Life Estate.** To protect Mark's right to continue to live in the house as long as he is able, and to protect it against creditors of his children, he can deed just a "remainder interest" in the house to his children (or to an irrevocable trust). This may be a better way to defeat the elective share, should Mark die before his wife. Since this is still a gift, the issue of whether this will affect Isabelle's eligibility must still be answered, based on the state rules.

- **Transfer House to Trust.** Mark can also transfer his entire interest in the house into an irrevocable trust. The advantage is that he can continue to control the house, by serving as sole trustee, yet protect it against creditors of his children. This may also be a good way to defeat the elective share, since after a period of time the general rule is that the property can no longer be counted as part of Mark's property for such purposes. Mark gave up ownership in the house on the date he deeded it into the trust. He can retain a right to live in the house for his lifetime, by putting that requirement right into the trust document. That can actually be useful for income tax purposes, since it will cause the basis of the house to be re-adjusted to the value as of Mark's death; that can save the children capital gains taxes when they go to sell the house after the father's death.

- **Sell House, Move in with Child**. See discussion under Study #2, above.

- **Plan for Mark.** Finally, no plan for a married couple is complete unless the possibility of *both* spouses needing long-term nursing home care is carefully considered and planned for. This study has focused only on obtaining Medicaid coverage for Isabelle; additional planning will also have to be done for Mark.

APPENDIX

The Importance of a Durable Power of Attorney

As soon as possible, the family member who is the potential nursing home resident—whether that is your spouse, parent or other family member—should sign a proper durable power of attorney. Without the power of attorney, should your family member become incompetent, there will be no one to sign documents or allow transfers and purchases for Medicaid planning purposes. Since the individual cannot sign, without the power of attorney you will be forced to hire a lawyer and seek appointment as the individual's guardian or conservator. Unfortunately, even with such appointment, you will need to have the approval of the judge in order to do any Medicaid planning-related transfers, and there is no guarantee you will get that approval. Some states actually have statutes that specifically authorize such transfers, but most do not. Since the primary purpose of the guardian/conservator is to protect the "ward" (i.e., the person who is under guardianship/conservatorship), the judge may be reluctant to permit transfers—even to family members—that will reduce or deplete the ward's assets.

Note that not just *any* durable power of attorney will do! The last thing you want to do is head out to your local office supply store for a $9.95 form, or purchase one (or obtain one for free) online. These basic forms will *not* contain the provisions you need to do Medicaid planning. For example, they rarely authorize gift giving and never mention Medicaid planning.

Even otherwise complete durable powers of attorney prepared by attorneys may not have the necessary Medicaid planning provisions. For example, they may omit the power to make gifts or may limit such gifts to the federal gift tax annual exclusion (currently $12,000 per person per year). Such a gift-giving limitation has its place in estate planning for the wealthy, but it can be severely limiting in a Medicaid planning context.

To be sure you have a power of attorney that will do what you need it to do, you really should hire an elder law attorney to prepare this document for you or your family member. Although the attorney's fee will be modest, it will certainly be more than the cost of the office supply form; however, it will be the best money you ever spent. With this properly prepared legal document, you will be able to make transfers to family members for Medicaid planning purposes without having to spend thousands of dollars going to court to be appointed a guardian or conservator, where you still risk having the judge turn down your request. Don't ignore the importance of this legal document!

Avoiding Non-attorney Assistance

A number of states have become plagued with non-attorney individuals or companies that aggressively market themselves as "Medicaid Estate Planners" or "Medicaid Asset Protection Specialists." By assisting the public with their Medicaid planning and applications, these non-attorneys may actually be engaging in the illegal "unauthorized practice of law." There have been several lawsuits shutting down some of the most egregious of these companies and individuals.

Too often the non-attorney individuals use inappropriate "Medicaid-friendly annuity" sales in order to quickly qualify their customers for Medicaid. Often there are more suitable options for the individual that are overlooked in favor of the annuity, which typically generates hefty commissions for the salesman while locking in the customer to an irrevocable and unchangeable investment or one with huge penalty fees if they decide to back out of it.

As you have certainly realized in reading this book, Medicaid planning is an extremely complicated area of the law. Do not trust your family's financial future to a non-lawyer who offers to quickly qualify your family member for Medicaid!

How to Find the Right Kind of Attorney

What you should not do: Open the Yellow Pages, look under "Attorneys," and pick one that says "Divorce/Corporate Law/Real Estate/Wills/Probate/Elder Law." There is simply no way one attorney can master all of these fields AND be competent in the specialized field of Medicaid planning.

What you should do: Locate an attorney who specializes in elder law, and particularly in Medicaid planning.

NAELA

A good place to start is at www.NAELA.org, which is the website for the National Association of Elder Law Attorneys (NAELA). Now just because somebody paid a few hundred dollars and joined this voluntary organization does not guarantee any degree of competence in Medicaid planning. The truth is that NAELA is open to any licensed attorney, no matter how much or how little experience he or she has. However, it is also true that just about any attorney who specializes in elder law, and who makes it a point to keep up with this rapidly changing area of the law, will be a member of NAELA. At a minimum, it shows that the attorney has an interest in this area of the law and it's a good place to start your search.

At www.NAELA.org, you can type in the zip code of the person for whom you are doing the planning. So if you live in Oregon, but you're concerned about your parents who reside in Massachusetts, then look for an attorney in Massachusetts, not Oregon. You want an attorney who is experienced with the laws, regulations, and local quirks of the state in which the person for whom you are doing the planning lives.

The NAELA listings offer the attorneys the opportunity to list their particular areas of specialty within elder law. For example, some elder law attorneys may enjoy the litigation side of elder law (i.e., going to court), and regularly handle conservatorship, guardianships, trust administration, probate cases, family battles, etc., but know little about Medicaid planning. On the other hand, an elder law attorney may be more concentrated on the estate planning side, with much tax knowledge and experience drafting complex wills and trusts, special needs trusts for disabled individuals, as well as Medicaid planning. Occasionally you'll find an elder law attorney who covers it all, or who at least works in a law firm that covers all of these related areas. Again, note that just because an attorney lists an area of specialty on the NAELA website does not guarantee the attorney is an expert in that area.

CELA Designation

There is one nationally recognized designation in the elder law field that actually means something. It is the "CELA" designation, which stands for "Certified Elder Law Attorney." Such designation is issued by the National Elder Law Foundation, and has the following requirements:

1) **Practice** - Attorney must have practiced law during the five years preceding his or her application and must still be practicing law.

2) **Integrity/Good Standing** - Attorney must be a member in good standing of the bars in all places in which he or she is licensed.

3) **Substantial Involvement** - Attorney must have spent an average of at least 16 hours per week practicing elder law during the three years preceding his or her application. In addition, he or she must have handled at least 60 elder law matters during those three years with a specified distribution among subjects as defined by the Foundation.

4) **Continuing Legal Education** - Attorney must have participated in at least 45 hours of continuing legal education in elder law during the preceding three years.

5) **Peer Review/Professional References** - Attorney must submit the names of five references from attorneys familiar with the attorney's competence and qualifications in elder law. These persons must themselves satisfy specified criteria.

6) **Examination** - Attorney must pass a full-day certification examination.

Note, however, that NOT having the CELA designation is not a black mark against the attorney. This designation is relatively recent, many attorneys have a busy practice already and don't want the hassle of sitting for an exam to obtain a designation they really don't need, and others may not have the broad experience in different facets of elder law, yet have a deep experience in the narrow area of Medicaid planning.

ACTEC

Another badge of expertise is membership in the American College of Trust and Estate Counsel (ACTEC). This "College" is not actually a school, but is a non-profit association composed of approximately 2,700 of the most accomplished estate planning practitioners in the United States and Canada. A lawyer cannot apply for membership in the College; Fellows of the College are nominated by other Fellows in their geographic area and are elected by the membership at large. To qualify for membership, a lawyer must have at least 10 years of experience in the active practice of probate and trust law or estate planning. Lawyers and law professors are elected to be Fellows by the other members, based on their outstanding professional reputation, exceptional skill, and substantial contributions to the field by lecturing, writing, teaching, and participating in bar activities. Historically, ACTEC attorneys have been considered the cream of the crop when it came to estate planning matters. However, recently some of them have extended their practice to include Medicaid planning as well.

Martindale-Hubbell®

Another measure of an attorney's expertise is his or her rating in Martindale-Hubbell®, the country's preeminent lawyer rating service. An AV® rating signifies a firm or attorney that has "achieved the highest levels of professional skill and integrity." The AV® rating is based on peer reviews by members of the Bar and Judiciary. That means that the lawyers and judges with whom the attorney has worked closely feel that the attorney is among the best in the business not only for his or her legal skills, but also for his or her honesty, integrity, and ethics. Attorney ratings can be found on the service's websites: www.martindale.com and www.lawyers.com.

State Certification

In recent years, many states have started to certify specialists in the law, such as bankruptcy, estate planning, litigation, divorce, etc. Some have also included the field of elder law as a specialty. Most states will piggyback on the national CELA certification requirements, so once again that's a pretty good indication that the attorney is committed to this area of the law.

Secrets to Finding an Expert

Here's what I do, when looking to find an expert in any area of the law, when I do not have personal knowledge: Go to the state bar association website and look for a list of current and past "CLE" ("continuing legal education") courses. Find one in the area of specialty you are interested in, and write down the names of all the attorneys who teach these courses. You can bet that the Bar Association will not let someone without a good reputation as an expert in the field be an instructor to other attorneys! You will also be able to review the listed attorneys' experience, since the brochures for these courses typically list a short professional bio of the attorney instructors.

In addition to the state bar association courses, there are also a number of national firms that produce CLE seminars for profit. Once again, they will have done the legwork for you, by checking around with other attorneys in your state for names of experts to serve as instructors. Two of the biggest producers of these kinds of seminars are the National Business Institute (NBI) and the Professional Education Seminar Institute (PESI). Check out their websites at www.NBI.com and www.PESI.com.

Who Is the Client?

Often family members other than or in addition to the potential Medicaid applicant will want to meet with the attorney. Although all family members generally want to save money if possible, some of the ways to do this may favor the younger generation at the expense of the older generation. Thus the elder law attorney must be careful to *identify who the client is.*

As a general rule, the person for whom the planning is being done, i.e., the potential Medicaid applicant and/or spouse, should be the client. This should be explained to all family members and also set out in a written fee agreement. The attorney will typically want to spend at least some time alone with the older generation to make sure that their wishes are fully understood and complied with. After all, *it is their money* that is the subject of the Medicaid planning, so they are the ones who should ultimately decide what they are comfortable doing or not doing.

For example, the attorney may come up with a recommendation that involves transferring 100% of the parent's money into an irrevocable trust. That may indeed be the best solution *on paper*, but it will leave the parent essentially impoverished and at the mercy of the trustee (who may or may not be the parent). The question must be asked: Is this the best option for the parent—or for the children? Sure, it offers the maximum protection of the parent's money, but at the expense of preventing the parent access to the parent's own funds! Thus, the children may lobby the parent to go along with this suggestion, since it is in the *children's* best interest, but the attorney must be careful that such planning is fully understood and agreed to by the parent.

Aggressive State Regulations

There is a trend among state legislatures to pass laws and/or issue regulations that are in clear violation of the federal Medicaid statutes. Apparently their approach is: "So sue me!" In other words, if an individual disagrees with the state's law or regulation, that individual can hire an attorney and sue the state, hoping to force a change or repeal of the illegal law or regulation. Of course, doing so forces the individual to spend thousands of dollars on legal fees, with no guarantee of a successful outcome (in some cases, the elderly client/plaintiff dies before the case has finished winding its way through the various levels of appeals within the legal system). The result is that the vast majority of residents of that state are required to give up legal rights and lose thousands of dollars in life savings, in order to comply with these illegal laws and regulations. The state knows this and is counting on this disparity in power to reduce the benefits it would otherwise have to pay out for its nursing home residents, thereby saving the state hundreds of thousands of dollars in Medicaid payments.

Note that even if a private attorney wanted to challenge the law or regulation for the benefit of all poor and elderly residents in his or her state, the attorney cannot do anything; in order to bring a legal action against the state in the hopes of changing the law or regulation, there must be an individual who is harmed as a result of the law or regulation. It takes a strong-willed and patient client—and one with deep pockets—who would be willing to be the plaintiff in a test case in the hopes of overturning the bad law or regulation.

Unfortunately, there is little the harmed individual resident can do under this system short of volunteering to be that test case.

2007 Figures

This book incorporates the 2007 federal figures for CSRA, MMMNA, etc.

The minimum MMMNA (currently $1,650) changes on July 1, 2007.

GLOSSARY

Agent: The person(s) who have legal authority to act on behalf of someone else, under a power of attorney document. *See* **Durable Power of Attorney**.

Annual Exclusion Gifts: Under federal gift tax laws, a certain amount of money or equivalent value assets may be gifted each year without requiring the filing of a federal gift tax return (Form 709). In 2006-7, this amount is $12,000 per gift recipient per year.

Attorney-in-fact: *See* **Agent**.

Basis: The purchase price of an asset, increased by certain transaction costs (and, for real estate, improvements). Used in calculating capital gains taxes.

CELA ("Certified Elder Law Attorney"): A designation offered by the National Elder Law Foundation to attorneys who have met certain requirements indicating both substantial experience and expertise in elder law and who pass an all-day exam.

Community Spouse: The spouse who resides in the community, when one spouse of a married couple is in the nursing home. Also known as the "healthy spouse."

Countable Asset: An asset owned by the Medicaid applicant (or spouse) that is counted for purposes of determining Medicaid eligibility.

CSRA ("Community Spouse Resource Allowance"): The amount of countable resources permitted to be owned by the Community Spouse, in order for the Institutionalized Spouse to qualify for Medicaid. In 2007 the maximum amount is $101,640 and the minimum amount is $20,328.

Domicile: A person's permanent residence and the place to which a person intends to return should he or she leave such place temporarily. Thus, a person may have multiple residences (i.e., homes in several states or countries) but only one domicile.

DRA: The Deficit Reduction Act of 2005, a federal law that was signed on February 8, 2006. This law changed the calculation of transfer penalties, lookback period, treatment of annuities, etc.

Durable Power of Attorney: A legal document where one person (the "principal") authorizes another person (the "agent" or "attorney-in-fact") to act on behalf of the first person. It can be either "limited" (the agent only has the specific powers listed in the document) or "general" (broad powers to do whatever the principal could have done had the principal been competent). "Durable" means that the agent will continue to have the power to act on behalf of the principal even if the principal becomes incompetent.

Estate Recovery: The legal process of a state to seek reimbursement from the "estate" of a deceased Medicaid recipient for all the money it spent on that recipient's care, while that person was receiving Medicaid. "Estate" for these purposes is defined in various ways by different states.

Excess Shelter Allowance: If the "shelter" costs of a Community Spouse exceed the shelter standard (i.e., 30% of the MMMNA: currently $495), then the **MMMNA** may be increased, up to the **maximum MMMNA,** by the amount of such excess. "Shelter" costs are limited to the following: rent or mortgage (including both principal and interest payments), real estate taxes, homeowner's insurance, condo or coop maintenance fees, and utility costs (either a state-set standard amount or actual costs, depending on the state rule).

Excluded Asset: An asset owned by a Medicaid applicant (or spouse) that is not counted for purposes of determining Medicaid eligibility. Also known as a **non-countable asset** or **exempt asset.**

Exempt Asset: *See* **Excluded Asset**.

Fair Hearing: An administrative appeal within the state agency that makes the determinations of financial eligibility for Medicaid applicants. It is usually an informal proceeding, but bringing an attorney is common.

Fraudulent Transfer: Also known as a fraudulent conveyance, such a transfer is one that is made by a debtor with actual intent to *hinder, delay, or defraud* any creditor of the debtor; or one that is made without receiving a reasonably equivalent value in exchange for the transfer, where the debtor was engaged or was about to engage in a transaction for which the remaining assets of the debtor were unreasonably small in relation to the transaction, or intended to incur, or believed or reasonably should have believed that he or she would incur, debts beyond his or her ability to pay as they became due. In short, someone making gifts in order to qualify for Medicaid could, in theory, have those gifts set aside and reversed by the state under this law, which is adopted in one form or another in all states. To date, this has not been invoked by states as a way to reverse Medicaid planning, but states may consider doing so at some point in the future.

Gifting Power: The specific authority in a **Durable Power of Attorney** to make gifts of your property to family members. This can be extremely valuable, allowing family members to do Medicaid planning for you even after you become incompetent. Unfortunately, most Powers of Attorney omit such authority.

Grantor: The person who creates and funds a trust.

HCBS ("Home and Community Based Services"): An optional state-provided Medicaid benefit to home-bound individuals who need nursing home level care.

Healthy Spouse: *See* **Community Spouse.**

Heirs: Those individuals entitled to receive a portion of a deceased person's probate estate upon such person's death, according to the laws of the person's state of domicile, if such person dies with no valid will.

Ill Spouse: *See* **Institutionalized Spouse.**

Institutionalized Spouse: The spouse who resides in the nursing home, when the other spouse of a married couple (i.e., the **Community Spouse**) is living in the community. Also referred to as the *nursing home spouse* or the *ill spouse*.

Inter Vivos Trust: A separate, stand-alone legal document that creates a trust. It is effective immediately upon signing. *See* **Testamentary Trust**.

Intestate: Dying without a will. In such case, the law of the state where the deceased person had his or her last permanent residence (**domicile**) will set forth how such property must be distributed.

Intestate Succession: The procedure of distributing the probate assets of a person who died with no will. See **Intestate**.

Irrevocable Trust: A trust that may not be revoked or amended by the creator of the trust.

Joint Tenancy with Right of Survivorship ("JTWROS"): Form of joint ownership of real estate where the interest of each owner passes automatically at death to the other (surviving) owner(s). *See* **Tenants in Common.**

Ladybird Deed: A deed that transfers the home to someone else, typically the transferor's children, while retaining the legal right to sell the house during the lifetime of the transferor, thereby avoiding probate. Not valid in all states.

Lien: A claim that is recorded in the registry of deeds office against a specific parcel of real estate, to ensure that the claim is satisfied before the real estate is sold. Title will not pass until the lien is released, so it is a way to guarantee that the property cannot be sold before satisfying the lien.

Life Estate: An interest in real estate that terminates upon the death of the owner of the interest. Until that time, the owner of the life estate has the right to the use and possession of the property and to the rents if it is rented out. *See* **Remainder Interest.**

Life Tenant: The owner of a life estate interest in a particular parcel of real estate. *See* **Remainder Interest.**

Living Trust: A trust that is created and operational during the lifetime of the creator. The term is usually used only to refer to a trust that is amendable and revocable by the creator. *See* **Testamentary Trust.**

Living Will: A legal document that states a person's wishes regarding termination of life support if the person has a terminal illness with no hope of recovery. Sometimes confused with a **living trust** because of the similar name, but it's completely different!

Lookback Period: The period of time prior to the date of a Medicaid application during which any gifts made by the person applying for Medicaid must be counted. Current lookback periods are 36 months for outright gifts made prior to February 8, 2006 and 60 months for all gifts made thereafter.

MMMNA ("The Minimum Monthly Maintenance Needs Allowance"): This is the minimum amount of income that a Community Spouse is entitled to have. If the Community Spouse has less than this amount, he or she is entitled to shift from the Institutionalized Spouse's income that amount of income necessary to increase the Community Spouse's income to the MMMNA. The MMMNA is set by the federal government and changes annually. The 2007 figure is $1,650 (changes on 7/1/07).

Maximum MMMNA: In certain cases, the **Community Spouse** may petition to increase his or her **MMMNA**, e.g., if the Community Spouse has high shelter-related costs or other unusual expenses, such as very high personal medical costs. If such costs are approved, the MMMNA can be increased to as high as $2,541 (2007 figure).

NAELA ("The National Academy of Elder Law Attorneys"): A national organization with membership limited to attorneys. It is the pre-eminent such organization, holding national conferences that assist the ongoing education of its members. (www.NAELA.org)

Non-countable Resource: *See* **Excluded Resource**

Penalty Divisor: The dollar number that is divided into the amount of a gift in order to determine the number of months of the **penalty period.** The divisor number varies from state to state and is typically updated annually to reflect the average monthly cost of a nursing home in the particular state (or region of the state, in some cases).

Penalty Period: The period of time during which an applicant for Medicaid coverage will be disqualified from such coverage, based on the amount of gifts made within the **lookback period.** *See* **Penalty Divisor.**

POD ("Pay On Death") Account: A bank account that is immediately transferred into the name of one or more named beneficiaries upon the death of the original owner of the account. It is used to avoid having to probate the bank account, thereby allowing immediate access to the funds in the account following the account owner's death.

Pooled Trust: A state chartered charitable organization specifically created to hold contributions of many disabled individuals, for the **supplemental needs** of each disabled individual. Each contribution is maintained in a separate account for the lifetime of the individual.

Power of Appointment: A power to change the distribution of trust assets from that which is set forth in the trust document. Such power may be exercised during the power-holder's lifetime or only following the power-holder's death (a so-called "testamentary power of appointment"). The trust document itself will set forth the conditions of exercise, e.g., must be exercised in the power-holder's will, etc.

Principal: The *principal* of a trust is the underlying assets titled in the name of the trust. Any interest, dividends, rent, etc., that are generated by these assets is called the trust *income*.

Probate Estate: The assets owned by an individual upon death that pass under the provisions of a will (or, if there is no will, by **intestate succession**). It includes all assets in the individual's sole name and excludes all assets that pass by right of survivorship (such as most jointly owned property) or beneficiary designation (such as life insurance, annuities, IRAs, 401(k)s, POD, TOD, etc.) or that are held in the name of a trust.

Remainder Beneficiary: Also known as *remainderman*. The individual who succeeds to the interest in real estate after the death of a person who owned a **life estate** in such property; also the individual who succeeds to an interest in a trust after the death of a prior beneficiary.

Remainder Interest: The interest in real estate that comes into the possession of the remainder beneficiaries upon the death of the owner of a **life estate.**

Example:

Mr. Smith owns Smith Farm. He deeds the farm to his children, reserving a **life estate**. The children have no rights to possession of the farm until Mr. Smith's death. Upon his death, all of the children own the farm equally. Thus, during Mr. Smith's lifetime, the children are the **remainder**

beneficiaries and own a **remainder interest** in the farm.

Resource: Any asset owned by a Medicaid applicant (or spouse), which is evaluated for purposes of determining Medicaid eligibility. Such resource may be **countable, unavailable,** or **excluded (exempt).**

Revocable Trust: A trust that may be revoked and amended at any time by the creator of the trust.

Self-Settled Trust: A trust funded with the assets of (and typically also created by) an individual for such individual's own benefit. *See* **Third-Party-Created Trust.**

Settlor: *See* **Grantor.**

Single: As used in this book, "single" means a person who was never married or who is divorced or widowed.

Special Needs Trust: A trust that is specifically created to distribute its assets for the benefit of a disabled individual in such a way that the trust will not disqualify the individual from receiving various government benefits. For these purposes, "special needs" are defined as those benefits and services that supplement but do not supplant, replace, or reduce otherwise available government benefits. Also known as a **Supplemental Needs Trust.**

Spend Down: The process of reducing the **countable assets** of a Medicaid applicant through various purchases and expenditures, so that the applicant will qualify for Medicaid coverage. The amount of excess assets is called the **spenddown** amount.

SSDI ("Social Security Disability Income"): A federal program that provides a minimal amount of income to individuals who are disabled as defined under the Social Security rules. Eligibility for these benefits is not based on the individual's income or assets.

SSI ("Supplemental Security Income"): A federal program that provides a minimal amount of income to individuals with very low assets and income. Many of the Medicaid asset and income rules are based on the SSI rules.

Supplemental Needs Trust: *See* **Special Needs Trust.**

Tangible Personal Property: Personal property that you can physically touch, such as furniture, a car, or jewelry. Thus, a stock or bond is not tangible personal property, because the paper it is printed on represents an ownership interest in something other than the actual piece of paper.

TEFRA Lien: A **lien** imposed on the residence of a Medicaid recipient during the recipient's lifetime to ensure that the house cannot be sold without first repaying the amount of Medicaid expenditures made by the state on behalf of the Medicaid recipient. This law was first enacted as part of the federal Tax Equity and Fiscal Responsibility Act ("TEFRA") of 1982. *See* **Lien.**

Tenants in Common: A form of joint ownership of real estate where, upon the death of each joint owner, such owner's percentage share of the property passes by the owner's will and not to the other joint owners. *See* **Joint Tenancy with Right of Survivorship.**

Tenants By the Entirety: A form of joint ownership of real estate where the only owners are a married couple. It offers some creditor protection to the spouses not available to non-spouses, in addition to the right of survivorship. It is not available in all states.

Testamentary Trust: A trust created within the provisions of a will. Thus, it only becomes effective following the death of the creator of the will.

Third-Party-Created Trust: A trust created and funded by someone other than the beneficiary or his or her spouse.

TOD ("Transfer On Death") Account: TOD accounts are available for most types of "paper" assets, such as savings and checking accounts in banks and credit unions, certificates of deposit, stocks, bonds, and other securities. Such accounts are immediately transferred into the name of a named beneficiary upon the death of the original owner. They are used to avoid having to probate the account or certificate and immediately pass title to the beneficiary following the original owner's death.

Transfer Without Fair Consideration: A gift. For example, selling one's house to one's children for $1 is really a gift of the full value of the house, less

$1. Such a transfer is without fair consideration, since the amount received by the seller was not the full value of the house.

Trust: A form of divided ownership: one person (the **trustee**) takes title to an asset for the benefit of another person (the beneficiary). It is essentially an agreement between the creator of the trust (known as the **grantor** or **settlor**) and the trustee, who oversees the trust property. The terms of the agreement are set forth in the trust document itself. A trust can be a free-standing, separate document (such as a **revocable trust** or **living trust** or **inter vivos trust**) or contained within the terms of a will (a **testamentary trust**).

Trustee: The individual or entity who manages and invests the trust assets and also determines the amount and frequency of distributions to the person or persons who benefit from such distributions (the beneficiaries of the trust). Many times family members serve as trustees for other family members, or a bank or trust company may be employed to do so.

Unavailable Resource: An asset that cannot be sold by the Medicaid applicant for legal reasons, e.g., an interest in an estate prior to distribution, an interest in ongoing litigation, etc.

ANNUITY (LIFE EXPECTANCY) TABLE

2001 Period Life Table, Social Security Administration
(Updated April 6, 2006)

Exact Age	Male Life Expectancy	Female Life Expectancy	Exact Age	Male Life Expectancy	Female Life Expectancy
50	27.85	31.75	76	9.29	11.33
51	27	30.85	77	8.77	10.71
52	26.16	29.95	78	8.27	10.11
53	25.32	29.07	79	7.78	9.52
54	24.5	28.18	80	7.31	8.95
55	23.68	27.31	81	6.85	8.4
56	22.86	26.44	82	6.42	7.87
57	22.06	25.58	83	6	7.36
58	21.27	24.73	84	5.61	6.88
59	20.49	23.89	85	5.24	6.42
60	19.72	23.06	86	4.89	5.98
61	18.96	22.24	87	4.56	5.56
62	18.21	21.43	88	4.25	5.17
63	17.48	20.63	89	3.97	4.81
64	16.76	19.84	90	3.7	4.47
65	16.05	19.06	91	3.45	4.15
66	15.36	18.3	92	3.22	3.86
67	14.68	17.54	93	3.01	3.59
68	14.02	16.8	94	2.82	3.35
69	13.38	16.07	95	2.64	3.13
70	12.75	15.35	96	2.49	2.93
71	12.13	14.65	97	2.35	2.75
72	11.53	13.96	98	2.22	2.58
73	10.95	13.28	99	2.11	2.43
74	10.38	12.62	100	2	2.29
75	9.83	11.97			

LIFE ESTATE TABLE (UNISEX)

Age	Life Estate	Remainder	Age	Life Estate	Remainder
50	0.84743	0.15257	76	0.50441	0.49559
51	0.83674	0.16126	77	0.48742	0.51258
52	0.82969	0.17031	78	0.47049	0.52951
53	0.82028	0.17972	79	0.45357	0.54643
54	0.81054	0.18946	80	0.43659	0.56341
55	0.80046	0.19954	81	0.41967	0.58033
56	0.79006	0.20994	82	0.40295	0.59705
57	0.77931	0.22069	83	0.38642	0.61358
58	0.76822	0.23178	84	0.36998	0.63002
59	0.75675	0.24325	85	0.35359	0.64641
60	0.74491	0.25509	86	0.33764	0.66236
61	0.73267	0.26733	87	0.32262	0.67738
62	0.72002	0.27998	88	0.30859	0.69141
63	0.70696	0.29304	89	0.29526	0.70474
64	0.69352	0.30648	90	0.28221	0.71779
65	0.6797	0.3203	91	0.26955	0.73045
66	0.66551	0.33449	92	0.25771	0.74229
67	0.65098	0.34902	93	0.24692	0.75308
68	0.6361	0.3639	94	0.23728	0.76272
69	0.62086	0.37914	95	0.22887	0.77113
70	0.60522	0.39478	96	0.22181	0.77819
71	0.58914	0.41086	97	0.21550	0.78450
72	0.57261	0.42739	98	0.21000	0.79000
73	0.55571	0.44429	99	0.20486	0.79514
74	0.53862	0.46138	100	0.19975	0.80025
75	0.52149	0.47851			

FEDERAL STATUTES

Here is a link to the federal statutes that govern Medicaid, as amended by the Deficit Reduction Act of 2005 (signed into law on February 8, 2006):

http://www.elderlawanswers.com/resources/DRA%20Integrated%203.doc

Note that even though the Medicaid program is created by these federal statutes, the states are given leeway in interpreting many of these sections, resulting in uncertainty and discrepancies from state to state.

If your state's own statutes, regulations or policies conflict with the federal law, an experienced elder law attorney will know whether to challenge the state in court and your likely chances of success. You should consider this option if the stakes in your personal situation are high enough.

- **42 U.S.C. § 1396p**—Liens, adjustments and recoveries, and transfers of assets.
  Here's where you'll find the rules governing gift penalty calculations, lookback periods, liens against your home, estate recovery after your death, annuities, and trusts.

- **42 USC 1396r-5**—Treatment of income and resources for certain institutionalized spouses.
  Sets forth the rules governing spouses, where one applies for Medicaid: Attribution of income and assets, MMMNA, CSRA, etc.

RESOURCES

1) www.NAELA.org: The main site of the National Academy of Elder Law Attorneys. Here's where you can search for an elder law attorney by zip code, specialty, etc.

2) Finding a good nursing home:
    a. www.medicare.gov/nursing/checklist.pdf: A great checklist of what to look for when selecting a nursing home.

    b. nccnhr.newc.com/uploads/NhConsumerGuide.pdf

    c. www.medicare.gov/Publications/Pubs/pdf/02174.pdf: Useful 64-page booklet on how to select a good nursing home.

    d. www.myziva.net: Help in choosing a nursing home.

    e. http://www.consumersunion.org/health/nursing-rpt603.htm: *Consumer Reports* article on nursing homes.

3) www.elderlawanswers.com: Information on elder law topics; resources; attorney lists; and a unique discussion forum where you can post questions and read others' answers.

4) www.senioranswers.org/Pages/cgs.sitemap.html: A great list of elder law links, sponsored by the Colorado Gerontological Society.

5) www.oasthook.com/legal information.php: A wonderful list of articles penned by this elder law firm, plus useful links.

6) www.brkdirect.com/spia/EZQUOTE.ASP: Use this site to calculate payments on immediate annuities.

7) http://www.njelderlaw.com/library listall typeup.asp: Several good articles on Medicaid planning, with examples.

8) www.BoulderElderLaw.com: Website of the author of this book; contains articles and info on Medicaid planning.

9) http://www.cms.hhs.gov/home/medicaid.asp: The main Medicaid page of the federal body that governs the Medicaid program, the Centers for Medicare and Medicaid Services ("CMS"). Here you can find detailed information on the Medicaid program, as well as links to relevant statutes, regulations, and agency letters.

10) www.healthlaw.org: Click on "Medicaid" for up-to-date articles.

11) https://s044a90.ssa.gov/apps10/poms.nsf/subchapterlist!openview&r estricttocategory=05011: Links to the various sections of the "POMS" (Social Security's *Program Operations Manual System*), which contain regulations and statutory policy interpretations that govern the Medicaid program.

12) Medicaid Annuities

    a. www.medicaidannuity.com: Krause Financial Services. Headed up by Dale Krause, who is an attorney, this company specializes in Medicaid annuities. Dale is very active with the elder law bar across the country and is obviously very knowledgeable about this area.

    b. www.osumrall.com: Sumrall & Associates.

STATE MEDICAID AGENCY CONTACTS

Alabama

Medicaid Agency of Alabama
501 Dexter Avenue
P.O. Box 5624
Montgomery, AL 36103-5624
Local: 1-334-242-5000
Toll free: 1-800-362-1504
Fax: 1-334-353-5989
Hours: 8:00am - 5:00pm
Web site: http://www.medicaid.state.al.us/

Alaska

Alaska Department of Health and Social Services
350 Main Street, Room 229
P.O. Box 110601
Juneau, AK 99811-0601
Local: 1-907-465-3355
Toll free: 1-800-780-9972
Fax: 1-907-465-3068
Hours: 8:00 am - 5:00 pm
Web site: http://www.hss.state.ak.us/dhcs

American Samoa

Department of Human Services of Hawaii
P.O. Box 339
Honolulu, HI 96809
Local: 1-808-587-3521
TTY: 1-808-692-7182
Hours: 7:45 am - 4:30 pm
Web site: http://www.med-quest.us/

Arizona

Health Care Cost Containment of Arizona
801 E. Jefferson
Phoenix, AZ 85034
Toll free: 1-800-526-3022 (national)
TTY: 1-602-417-4191
Spanish: 1-602-417-7700
Fax: 1-602-252-2136
Hours: 7am-9pm M-F; 8-6 Sat
Web site: http://www.ahcccs.state.az.us

Arkansas

Department of Human Services of Arkansas
P.O. Box 1437, Slot 1100
Donaghey Plaza South
Little Rock, AR 72203-1437
Local: 1-501-682-8233
Toll free: 1-800-482-5431
TTY: 1-501-682-6789
Spanish: 1-800-482-8988
Fax: 1-501-682-1197
E-mail: Delores.Pinkerton@medicaid.state.ar.us
Hours: 8:00 am - 4:30 pm
Web site: http://www.medicaid.state.ar.us/

California

California Department of Health Services
P.O. Box 997413
Sacramento, CA 95899-7413
Local: 1-916-636-1980
Fax: 1-916-552-9425
Hours: 8AM-5PM
Web site: www.medi-cal.ca.gov

Colorado

Department of Health Care Policy and Financing
1570 Grant Street
Denver, CO 80203-1818
Local: 1-303-866-2993
Toll free: 1-800-221-3943
TTY: 1-303-866-3883
Spanish: 1-303-866-1416
Fax: 1-303-866-4411
Hours: 8:00 am - 5:00 pm
Web site: http://www.chcpf.state.co.us

Connecticut

Department of Social Services of Connecticut
25 Sigourney Street
Hartford, CT 06106-5033
Local: 1-860-424-4908
Toll free: In-State Calls Only 1-800-842-1508
Fax: 1-860-951-9544
E-mail: pgr.dss@po.state.ct.us
Hours: 8:00 am - 5:00 pm
Web site: http://www.dss.state.ct.us

Delaware

Delaware Health and Social Services
1901 N. DuPont Highway
P.O. Box 906, Lewis Bldg.
New Castle, DE 19720
Local: 1-302-255-9500
Toll free: 1-800-372-2022
Fax: 1-302-255-9469
E-mail: dhssinfo@state.de.us
Hours: 8:00 am - 4:30 pm
Web site: www.state.de.us/dhss/index.html

Florida

Agency for Health Care Administration of Florida
P.O. Box 13000, Tallahassee, FL 32317-3000
Local: 1-850-488-3560
Toll free: In-State Calls Only 1-866-762-2237
Fax: 1-850-488-2520
Hours: 8:00 am - 5:00 pm ET
Web site: www.fdhc.state.fl.us/

Georgia

Georgia Department of Community Health
2 Peachtree Street, NW, Atlanta, GA 30303
Local: 1-770-570-3300
Toll free: 1-866-322-4260
Fax: 1-270-804-7442
Hours: 8:00 am - 5:00 pm
Web site: ghp.georgia.gov

Hawaii

Department of Human Services of Hawaii
P.O. Box 339, Honolulu, HI 96809
Local: 1-808-587-3521
TTY: 1-808-692-7182
Hours: 7:45 am - 4:30 pm
Web site: http://www.med-quest.us/

Idaho

Idaho Department of Health and Welfare
3232 Elder, Boise, ID 83705-4711
Local: 1-208-334-5747
Toll free: 1-877-200-5441
TTY: 1-208-332-7205
Fax: 1-208-364-1888
Hours: 8 am - 5 pm
Web site: http://www2.state.id.us/dhw/medicaid/

Illinois

Illinois Department of Healthcare and Family Services
201 South Grand Avenue, East
Springfield, IL 62763
Local: 1-217-782-1200
Toll free: 1-866-468-7543
Spanish: 1-217-785-8036
E-mail: hfswebmaster@illinois.gov
Hours: 8:00 am - 4:45 pm CT
Web site: http://www.hfs.illinois.gov/

Indiana

Family and Social Services Administration of Indiana
402 W. Washington Street
P.O. Box 7083
Indianapolis, IN 46207-7083
Local: 1-317-233-4455
Toll free: 1-800-889-9949
Spanish: 1-317-234-0225
Fax: 1-317-232-7382
Hours: 8:00 am - 4:30 pm
Web site: http://www.in.gov/fssa/healthcare/

Iowa

Department of Human Services of Iowa
Hoover State Office Building
5th Floor
Des Moines, IA 50319-0114
Local: 1-515-327-5121
Toll free: 1-800-338-8366
Fax: 1-515-281-4597
Hours: 12:00 pm - 4:00 pm CT M-F

Kansas

Department of Social and Rehabilitation Services
915 SW Harrison Street
Topeka, KS 66612
Local: 1-785-274-4200
Toll free: 1-800-766-9012
TTY: 1-785-296-1491
Fax: 1-785-296-2173
Hours: 8:00 am-5:00 pm(CST)
Web site: http://www.srskansas.org/hcp/

Kentucky

Cabinet for Health Services of Kentucky
P.O. Box 2110
Frankfort, KY 40602-2110
Local: 1-502-564-4321
Toll free: 1-800-635-2570
Fax: 1-502-226-1898
Hours: 8:00 am - 4:30 pm
Web site: www.chfs.ky.gov

Louisiana

Louisiana Department of Health and Hospital
P.O. Box 91278
Baton Rouge, LA 70821-9278
Local: 1-225-342-5774
Toll free: In-State Calls Only 1-888-342-6207
TTY: 1-225-216-7387
Spanish: 1-225-219-0214
Fax: 1-225-342-9508
E-mail: thomascollins@dhhmail.dhh.state.la.us.gov
Hours: 8:00 am - 4:30 pm
Web site: www.medicaid.dhh.louisiana.gov

Maine

Maine Department of Health and Human Services
442 Civic Center Drive
11 State House Station
Augusta, ME 04333-0011
Local: 1-207-624-7539 (Eligibility)
Toll free: 1-800-977-6740 (option 2)
TTY: 1-207-287-1828
Fax: 1-207-287-9229
Hours: 8:00 am - 5:00 pm
Web site: www.state.me.us/bms

Maryland

Department of Health and Mental Hygiene
P.O. Box 17259
Baltimore, MD 21203-7259
Local: 1-410-767-5800
Toll free: 1-800-492-5231
Fax: 1-410-333-7141
E-mail: dhrhelp@dhr.state.md.us
Hours: 8:00 am - 5:00 pm
Web site: www.dhmh.state.md.us

Massachusetts

Office of Health and Human Services of Massachusetts
600 Washington Street
Boston, MA 02111
Local: 1-617-628-4141 (for provider only)
Toll free: 1-800-325-5231
Fax: 1-617-210-5820
E-mail: mainquiries@unisys.com
Hours: 8:00 am - 5:00 pm
Web site: www.mass.gov/masshealth

Michigan

Michigan Department of Community Health
Sixth Floor, Lewis Cass Building
320 South Walnut Street
Lansing, MI 48913
Local: 1-517-373-3740
Toll free: In-State Calls Only 1-800-642-3195
Fax: 1-517-335-5007
Hours: 8:00 am - 5:00 pm M-F
Web site: www.michigan.gov/mdch

Minnesota

Department of Human Services of Minnesota
444 Lafayette Road North
St. Paul, MN 55155
Local: 1-651-297-3933
Toll free: 1-800-333-2433
TTY: 1-651-296-5705
Fax: 1-651-296-5690
Hours: 8:00 am - 4:30 pm
Web site: http://www.dhs.state.mn.us/

Mississippi

Office of the Governor of Mississippi
239 North Lamar Street, Suite 801
Robert E. Lee Bldg.
Jackson, MS 39201-1399
Local: 1-601-359-6050
Toll free: 1-800-421-2408
Fax: 1-601-359-6048
E-mail: exrcc@medicaid.state.ms.us
Hours: 7:30 am-5:00 pm
Web site: http://www.dom.state.ms.us/

Missouri

Department of Social Services of Missouri
221 West High Street
P.O. Box 1527
Jefferson City, MO 65102-1527
Local: 1-573-751-4815
Toll free: In-State Calls Only 1-800-392-2161
Fax: 1-573-751-6564
Hours: 8:00 am - 5:00 pm
Web site: www.dss.mo.gov/dms

Montana

Montana Department of Public Health & Human Services-Division
of Child and Adult Health Resources
1400 Broadway, Cogswell Building
P.O. Box 8005
Helena, MT 59604-8005
Local: 1-406-444-4540
Toll free: In-State Calls Only 1-800-362-8312
Fax: 1-406-444-2547
E-mail: dphhstech@state.mt.us
Hours: 8:00 am - 5:00 pm MT
Web site: http://www.dphhs.mt.gov

Nebraska

Nebraska Department of Health and Human Services System
P.O. Box 95044
Lincoln, NE 68509-5044
Local: 1-402-471-3121
Toll free: 1-800-430-3244
TTY: 1-402-471-9570
Fax: 1-402-471-9449
E-mail: Mike.Harris@hhss.state.ne.us
Hours: 8:00 am - 5:00 pm
Web site: www.hhs.state.gov

Nevada

Nevada Department of Human Resources,
Division for Aging Services
1100 East William Street
Suite 101
Carson City, NV 89701
Local: 1-775-684-7200
Fax: 1-775-687-3893
Hours: 7:30 am – 5 pm M-F for all
Web site: www.nvaging.net/

New Hampshire

New Hampshire Department of Health and Human Services
129 Pleasant Street
Concord, NH 03301-3857
Local: 1-603-271-4322
Toll free: In-State Calls Only 1-800-852-3345 x8166
Fax: 1-603-271-4643
Hours: 8:00 am - 4:30 pm
Web site: http://www.dhhs.state.nh.us

New Jersey

Department of Human Services of New Jersey
Quakerbridge Plaza, Building 7
P.O. Box 712
Trenton, NJ 08625-0712
Local: 1-609-588-2600
Toll free: In-State Calls Only 1-800-356-1561
Spanish: 1-800-356-1561
Fax: 1-609-588-3583
E-mail: mahs.response@dhs.state.nj.us
Hours: 8:00 am - 5:00 pm
Web site: www.state.nj.us/humanservices/dmahs

New Mexico

Department of Human Services of New Mexico
Areas Covered: NM
P.O. Box 2348Santa Fe, NM 87504-2348
Local: 1-505-827-3100
Toll free: 1-888-997-2583
TTY: 1-505-827-3184
Spanish: 1-800-432-6217
Fax: 1-505-827-3185
Hours: 8:00 am - 5:00 pm
Website: http://www.state.nm.us/hsd/mad

New York

New York State Department of Health, Office of Medicaid Management
Governor Nelson A. Rockefeller Empire State Plaza, Corning Tower Building
Albany, NY 12237
Local: 1-518-486-9057
Toll free: 1-800-541-2831
Fax: 1-518-486-6852
E-mail: medicaid@health.state.ny.us
Hours: 8:00 am - 4:45 pm
Web site: http://www.health.state.ny.us/

North Carolina

North Carolina Department of Health and Human Services
Division of Medical Assistance
2501 Mail Service Center
Raleigh, NC 27699-2501
Local: 1-919-855-4100
TTY: 1-877-733-4851
Spanish: 1-919-855-4400
Fax: 1-919-733-6608
E-mail: care.line@ncmail.net
Hours: 8:00AM-5:00PM
Web site: http://www.dhhs.state.nc.us/dma/

North Dakota

Department of Human Services of North Dakota - Medical Services
600 E. Boulevard Avenue
Bismarck, ND 58505-0250
Local: 1-701-328-2321
Toll free: 1-800-755-2604
TTY: 1-701-328-8950
Fax: 1-701-328-1060
E-mail: sogaph@state.nd.us
Hours: 8:00 am - 5:00 pm
Web site: www.state.nd.us/humanservices

Northern Mariana Islands

Department of Public Health Commonwealth of the Northern
Mariana Islands
P.O. Box 409 CK
Saipan, MP 96950
011-670-234-8950 ext. 2905

Ohio

Department of Job and Family Services of Ohio - Ohio Health Plans
30 East Broad Street
31st Floor
Columbus, OH 43215-3414
Local: 1-614-728-3288
Toll free: 1-800-324-8680
Fax: 1-614-752-3986
Hours: 7 am - 8 pm/Sat-Sun 8-5
Web site: http://jfs.ohio.gov/ohp

Oklahoma

Health Care Authority of Oklahoma
4545 N. Lincoln Boulevard
Suite 124
Oklahoma City, OK 73105
Local: 1-405-522-7171 (also (405) 522-7300)
Toll free: 1-800-522-0310
TTY: 1-405-522-7179
Fax: 1-405-522-7100
Hours: 7:30am - 5:30pm
Web site: www.okohca.org

Oregon

Oregon Department of Human Services
500 Summer Street, NE
3rd Floor
Salem, OR 94310-1014
Local: 1-503-945-5772
Toll free: In-State Calls Only 1-800-527-5772
TTY: 1-503-945-5895
Fax: 1-503-373-7689
Hours: 8:00 am - 5:00 pm
Web site: oregon.gov/dhs/index.shtml

Pennsylvania

Department of Public Welfare of Pennsylvania
Health and Welfare Building, Rm 515
P.O. Box 2675
Harrisburg, PA 17105
Local: 1-717-787-1870
Toll free: 1-800-692-7462
TTY: 1-717-705-7103
Hours: 8:30am - 4:45pm
Web site: www.dpw.state.pa.us/omap/dpwomap.asp

Puerto Rico

Medicaid Office of Puerto Rico and Virgin Islands
GPO Box 70184
San Juan, PR 00936
Local: 1-787-725-4300
Toll free: 1-877-725-4300
Fax: 1-787-759-8179
Hours: 8:00 am - 4:30 pm

Rhode Island

Department of Human Services of Rhode Island
Louis Pasteur Building
600 New London Avenue
Cranston, RI 02921
Local: 1-401-462-5300
Toll free: In-State Calls Only 1-800-984-8989
TTY: 1-401-462-3363
Fax: 1-401-521-4875
Hours: 8:30 am - 4:00 pm
Web site: www.dhs.ri.gov

South Carolina

South Carolina Department of Health and Human Services
P.O. Box 8206
Columbia, SC 29202-8206
Local: 1-803-898-2500
Toll free: 1-888-549-0820
Fax: 1-803-898-4515
E-mail: info@dhhs.state.sc.us
Hours: 8:00 am - 5:00 pm M-Th
Web site: http://www.dhhs.state.sc.us

South Dakota

Department of Social Services of South Dakota
700 Governors Drive
Richard F Kneip Bldg.
Pierre, SD 57501
Local: 1-605-773-3495
Toll free: In-State Calls Only 1-800-452-7691
Spanish: 1-800-305-9673
Fax: 1-605-773-5246
E-mail: MedElig@state.sd.us
Hours: 8:00 am - 5:00 pm
Web site: www.state.sd.us/social/medical

Tennessee

Bureau of TennCare
310 Great Circle Rd.
Nashville, TN 37243
Toll free: 1-866-311-4287
Fax: 1-615-741-0882
Hours: 7:00am - 6:00 pm
Web site: http://state.tn.us/tenncare

Texas

Health and Human Services Commission of Texas
4900 N. Lamar Boulevard
4th Floor
Austin, TX 78701
Local: 1-512-424-6500
Toll free: In-State Calls Only 1-877-541-7905
TTY: 1-512-407-3250
E-mail: medicaid@hhsc.state.tx.us
Hours: 7:30 am - 5:30 pm
Web site: http://www.hhsc.state.tx.us

Utah

Utah Department of Health
288 North 1460 West
P.O. Box 143101
Salt Lake City, UT 84114-3101
Local: 1-801-538-6155
Toll free: 1-800-662-9651
Spanish: 1-800-662-9651
Fax: 1-801-538-6805
Hours: 8:00 am - 5:00 pm
Web site: http://health.utah.gov/medicaid/

Vermont

Agency of Human Services of Vermont
103 South Main Street
Waterbury, VT 05676-1201
Local: 1-802-879-5900
Toll free: In-State Calls Only 1-800-250-8427
TTY: 1-802-241-1282
Fax: 1-802-241-2897
Hours: 8:00 am - 4:30 pm
Web site: www.ovha.state.vt.us

Virgin Islands

Medicaid Office of Puerto Rico and Virgin Islands
GPO Box 70184
San Juan, PR 00936
Local: 1-787-725-4300
Toll free: 1-877-725-4300
Fax: 1-787-759-8179
Hours: 8:00 am - 4:30 pm

Virginia

Department of Medical Assistance Services
600 East Broad Street
Suite 1300
Richmond, VA 23219
Local: 1-804-786-7933
Fax: 1-804-225-4512
E-mail: comm@dss.state.va.us
Hours: 8:30 am - 4:30 pm ET
Web site: www.dmas.virginia.gov

Washington

Department of Social and Health Services of Washington
P.O. Box 45505
Olympia, WA 98504-5505
Local: 1-800-562-6188
Toll free: In-State Calls Only 1-800-562-3022
Fax: 1-360-586-1209
Hours: 7:30 am - 4:30 pm
Web site: www.adsa.dshs.wa.gov

Washington, D.C.

DC Healthy Family
825 North Capitol Street, NE
5th Floor
Washington, DC 20002
Local: 1-202-742-5506
Toll free: 1-888-557-1116
TTY: 1-202-639-4041
Fax: 1-202-610-3209
Hours: 8:15 am - 4:45 pm EST
Web site: http://dchealth.dc.gov/index.asp

West Virginia

West Virginia Department of Health & Human Resources
350 Capitol Street
Room 251
Charleston, WV 25301-3709
Local: 1-304-558-1700
Fax: 1-304-558-2515
E-mail: medman@wvdhhr.org
Hours: 8am - 5pm M-F
Web site: http://www.wvdhhr.org/bms/

Wisconsin

Wisconsin Department of Health and Family Services
1 West Wilson Street
P.O. Box 309
Madison, WI 53701-0309
Local: 1-608-221-5720
Toll free: 1-800-362-3002
TTY: 1-608-267-7371
Fax: 1-608-221-8815
E-mail: webmaster@dhfs.state.wi.us
Hours: 7:00 am - 5:00 pm
Web site: www.dhfs.state.wi.us/medicaid/index.htm

Wyoming

Wyoming Department of Health
147 Hathaway Building
Cheyenne, WY 82002
Local: 1-307-777-7531
TTY: 1-307-777-5648
Fax: 1-307-777-6974
E-mail: iolesk@state.wy.us
Hours: 8:00 am - 5:00 pm MT
Web site: www.healthywyoming.org

MEDICAID QUESTIONNAIRES

Before you meet with an elder law attorney, you should pull together all relevant financial and family information. An example of what information is typically needed to make your meeting with your attorney as productive as possible is listed here.

1) QUESTIONNAIRE FOR A SINGLE PERSON:
   (divorced, widowed or never married)

   Go to www.BoulderElderLaw.com

   a. Click **Medicaid Planning** in the left menu

   b. Click Medicaid Questionnaires for Download in the left menu

   c. Click Medicaid Planning Questionnaire for a *Single Individual*

   d. Open the pdf file on your screen and print out the document on your printer

2) QUESTIONNAIRE FOR A MARRIED COUPLE:

   Go to www.BoulderElderLaw.com

   a. Click **Medicaid Planning** in the left menu

   b. Click Medicaid Questionnaires for Download in the left menu

   c. Click Medicaid Planning Questionnaire for a *Married Couple*

   d. Open the pdf file on your screen and print out the document on your printer

INDEX

Updates and Corrections

Writing a book on a legal topic is like trying to hit a moving target! In between new editions of this book, you will be entitled to free updates as part of the cost of the book.

(If you find any errors, please let us know. To thank you for your trouble, we'll give you credit on the Updates webpage.)

Go to **www.MedicaidSecrets.com/updates** frequently to check for:

- changes in federal and state laws that affect Medicaid planning;
- changes in state regulations that affect the interpretation of the law;
- new planning techniques and ideas;
- new tips and practical applications of the ideas in the book; and
- new resources, articles, and websites of interest to readers of this book.

Feedback Wanted

We want your comments and feedback!

If there is anything in the book that was difficult to understand, anything you particularly liked, any topics you wish to see covered in a future edition, any typos you spotted, etc., please send us an email at feedback@MedicaidSecrets.com. Thank you!

Printed in the United States
75451LV00005B/205-345